A PATIENT'S GUIDE TO UNNECESSARY KNEE SURGERY

"Everyone needs to read this book to avoid unnecessary surgery. Dr. Grelsamer's writing style makes this an easy useful read with easily retained knowledge."

—Lewis G. Maharam, MD, FACSM, aka Running Doc,
past president of GNYRC American College of Sports Medicine

"Dr. Grelsamer's book will help patients navigate the confusing and at times conflicting advice given by doctors about knee injuries and their treatment. His advice is timely, easy to understand, and laced with humor and wit. Along the way he gives advice on how to keep your knees happy and healthy."

—Elizabeth Arendt, MD

"After reading this book, my first reaction was: Amen! Not the automatic prayer response, but in a true sense of affirmation and agreement. Dr. Grelsamer relies on his broad and deep experience to 'tell it like it is' in a style and language that anyone can understand. He writes with honesty, integrity, humor, and yes, a wisdom that comes with a few gray hairs. It is rare for two orthopedic surgeons to agree in detail with one another, but this is one of those occasions. This book needed to be written, and I am happy that Dr. Grelsamer had the drive (and guts) to see it through. I enthusiastically recommend this book to anyone who has a knee—if it doesn't hurt now, the odds are it will. It should also be required reading for all med students, primary care docs, and especially first-year orthopedic residents."

—Alan Merchant, MD

"Dr. Grelsamer's comprehensive and authoritative book, *A Patient's Guide to Unnecessary Knee Surgery* is a must read for anyone contemplating knee surgery. Dr. Grelsemer summarizes some of the most common problems we see with regard to misdiagnosis and unnecessary surgery and he does it in an 'easy to read' fashion, making this topic understandable to all laypersons. Grelsemer makes this part of orthopedics approachable and allows readers to understand what was once only known to those of us in the field. Many injuries require surgery, however, many do not. It is imperative to understand which category your knee problem falls into so that patients don't make decisions from a place of pain (when most of us will do anything to get out of it)."

—Beth Shubin-Stein, MD

"In *A Patient's Guide to Unnecessary Knee Surgery*, Dr. Grelsamer has assembled a wealth of practical knowledge for patients who find themselves with a knee problem and don't know where to start looking for answers. In this age of the internet, there is a vast amount of unfiltered information and misinformation on the web. Most commercial websites have a commercial incentive for their information. Patients sense this bias and next turn to family and friends who have often unknowingly accepted portions of the misinformation. With the changes in medicine, the friendly local family physician is often no longer in the loop and the patient thus presents directly to a knee specialist that they often select with limited guidance from the web or insurance listing. Dr. Grelsamer points out that while the vast majority of orthopedic surgeons are well meaning and well-trained and would agree with the information is this *Patient's Guide*, a minor number either lack knowledge for the patient's specific problem or less so, may be motivated by a goal of surgical volume. Thus, caveat emptor unfortunately still applies in medicine today: "the principle that the buyer alone is responsible for checking the quality and suitability of goods before a purchase is made," per Google search in 2016. *Patient's Guide* allows a patient to become educated to the level of asking appropriate questions of their knee surgeon and even offers non-operative options to consider in the initial stages of their journey to knee happiness. As a practicing knee subspecialist, I would enjoy consulting with patients who have read the *Patient's Guide*. We could spend the consultation time discussing my recommendations based on the current world literature—avoiding the time necessary to educate patients about knee terminology, MRI limitations, and the fact that a vast majority of knee problems have nonsurgical solutions. This book affords patients a well-rounded discussion of treatment options, and allows them to become fully informed—the key to moving forward together with their knee doctor."

—Jack Farr, MD

"Dr. Grelsamer has written the comprehensive and honest guide for patients who have knee problems. His book should be a 'must read' for all who have experienced knee problems and for anyone who plans to see a knee specialist for evaluation and treatment."

—Phillip Bauman, MD

A PATIENT'S GUIDE TO UNNECESSARY KNEE SURGERY

How to Avoid the Pitfalls of Hasty Medical Advice

Ronald P. Grelsamer, MD

Skyhorse Publishing

Skyhorse Publishing books may be purchased in bulk at special discounts for sales promotion, corporate gifts, fund-raising, or educational purposes. Special editions can also be created to specifications. For details, contact the Special Sales Department, Skyhorse Publishing, 307 West 36th Street, 11th Floor, New York, NY 10018 or info@skyhorsepublishing.com.

Visit our website at www.skyhorsepublishing.com.

10 9 8 7 6 5 4 3 2

Library of Congress Cataloging-in-Publication Data is available on file.

Cover design by Tom Lau
Cover photo credit iStockphoto

Print ISBN: 978-1-5107-1687-2
Ebook ISBN: 978-1-5107-1689-6

Printed in the United States of America

To my wife Sharon whose patience made this book possible, and to Frank Stinchfield, MD who taught me to treat each patient like a friend.

CONTENTS

Acknowledgments xi
Introduction xiii

Chapter 1 Why Doctors Sometimes Misinform You 1

Chapter 2 The Misleading MRI 7

Chapter 3 Life-Threatening Torn Cartilage 21

Chapter 4 Stamp Out Torn Ligaments 43

Chapter 5 "Urgent" Arthritis Surgery 75

Chapter 6 The Hidden Causes of Knee Pain: Part I—Your Kneecap: Chondromalacia, Patellofemoral Syndrome 105

Chapter 7 The Hidden Causes of Knee Pain—Part 2 133

Chapter 8 Does Anyone Here Know How To Take an X-Ray? 145

Chapter 9 The Placebo: A Misunderstood Treatment 155

Chapter 10 Injuring Your Knee in the Name of Health 165

Chapter 11 Exercises for a Healthy Knee 175

Chapter 12 Personal Injury and the Law 195

Chapter 13 How to Find the Right Knee Doctor 203

Chapter 14 Should You Have Surgery in an Outpatient Surgery Center? 211

Index 213
About the Author 217

Acknowledgments

Thanks first and foremost to my wife Sharon and to my children Dominique and Marc who have put up with the time involved in putting this book together.

Thanks to my patients for proving me correct in believing that people are increasingly looking to be educated.

Thanks to Steven Arnold, MD for his help with Chapter 13.

Finally, thanks to my colleagues with suspect scruples without whom there would have been no need for this book.

Introduction

The wheel turns.

When this book was first published in 2002 under the title *What Your Doctor May NOT Tell You About Knee Pain and Surgery*, I expected to get hate mail from my colleagues; but at least the book would serve as a wake-up call to those suffering from knee pain and those paying for it.

Nothing of the kind happened.

I received a few letters from colleagues saying they wished they themselves had written the book, and doctors in other medical disciplines contacted me to point out similar issues in their own specialty.

A major television network was most interested in producing a piece based on that book; but in the end, disbelief won out. The message was watered down to a simple "get a second opinion."

We are now well into the twenty-first century, and the cost and delivery of health care have moved up a few notches in our consciousness.

The time is ripe to revisit the subject.

As the sixties saying goes, "If you're not part of the solution, you're part of the problem." If you don't speak up when you see something wrong, you are partly responsible for the persistence of that wrong.

Many people get bad advice when it comes to their knee. I would like to think that this book can help right this wrong.

Know that most everything you will read in this text falls into the category of mainstream orthopedics; there is nothing extreme here. This not an alternative medicine book. All concepts put forth here can be found in orthopedic textbooks and in the most prestigious orthopedic journals. The need for this book comes from the fact that the *public perception* of knee care is at variance with the truth. The misinformation is perpetuated by practitioners who are incompletely educated about knee issues and/or shamelessly unscrupulous.

When I entered practice more than thirty years ago, I thought the issues outlined in this book would correct themselves in rapid order. How could such miscarriages of medical care and justice continue? Yet, nothing has changed—at least not for the better. The exaggerated reliance on tests such as MRIs is getting worse, and there appears to be more unnecessary surgery than ever before.

After reading this book you should be better able to recognize bad advice when you see it, and you should be better able to take care of your knee—both before and after it starts to hurt. In short, this book is intended to help you take control of your knee care.

Note: *The knee surgery referred to here is outpatient surgery, namely arthroscopic surgery, not knee replacement surgery. That said, a number of traditional inpatient procedures (including knee replacements) are gradually being shifted to outpatient settings in freestanding surgical centers, and this is discussed in Chapter 13.*

CHAPTER 1

Why Doctors Sometimes Misinform You

I am very proud of the orthopedic profession. Going back over one hundred years—and especially over the last fifty—orthopedic innovations have vastly improved our quality of life. There are hip replacements, knee replacements, fracture surgeries, arthroscopies, scoliosis correction; the list goes on and on.

For the most part of course, doctors are earnest, intelligent, and knowledgeable, and they are dedicated to making people feel better. For the most part.

Alas, there also exists a being I call the LK-SS doctor: Limited Knowledge-Suspect Scruples Doctor.

> <u>Limited Knowledge</u>: It seems incredible that after four years of medical school and four to six more years of orthopedic training, an orthopedist or physiatrist (rehabilitation specialist) could still be deficient in his or her knowledge of the knee. And yet it's true. Over the last five decades, the world of orthopedics has dramatically expanded.

When I was in training in the early 1980s, some of my teachers had had no formal training in orthopedic surgery (orthopedic surgery being the surgery of bones and joints). They had trained as general surgeons and somewhere along the line had taken an interest in orthopedics. Up until the 1960s, the sum total of orthopedic knowledge was small enough to allow this. General surgeons, for example, routinely set fractures.

The field became more sophisticated. A different approach was developed for every type of fracture in each bone; controversies developed around each of these fractures. The world of fractures became a field unto itself that could no longer be considered a small surgical aside. Techniques were also perfected for spinal deformities, arthritis, sports trauma, and pediatric conditions. These operations became too numerous and complex for a general surgeon to simply pick up in his spare time. By the 1980s, surgeons who had taken specialty training in orthopedic surgery were addressing most of the orthopedic conditions treated in the United States.

Incredibly, orthopedics evolved into a yet more complicated field, each part of the body becoming a specialty unto itself. Consider the scientific literature: there are at least two English-language journals dealing only with knees, many journals dealing with sports injuries, entire journals devoted to the hand, to the shoulder, to the spine, to *only* the foot, to joint replacements, to fractures, or to children's orthopedics.

People were amazed in the 1970s when an entire book was devoted to the knee. Now, even the knee is nearly too large a subject. I have written a medical textbook dealing exclusively with the kneecap—and there are now at least five on the subject.

A medical school curriculum calls for, at the very most, one or two weeks of orthopedic training sandwiched in between the "more important" subjects. With occasional exceptions, medical students know next to nothing about orthopedics when they graduate.

An orthopedist in training is already an MD and is called a resident. He or she learns the basics pertaining to each part of the body and learns how to perform the most common procedures. All orthopedists learn to recognize and treat fractures. However, the world of orthopedics is too large for an orthopedist out of general training to know all there is to know about hands, feet, knees, shoulders, and so forth. So orthopedists often now do fellowships to hone their skills in a specific area. There are hand fellowships, spine fellowships, and so forth. There are very few comprehensive knee fellowships because the world of knee surgery has been split into two parts. In the early to mid-1970s, the new field of knee replacement surgery fell into the orbit of hip replacement surgery that preceded it by a number of years. Surgeons proficient in hip replacement surgery performed most of the knee replacements. On the other hand, knee arthroscopies and ligament reconstructions were first performed in the early 1980s by self-titled sports orthopedists. Therefore there exist knee joint replacement surgeons (and fellowships), as well as knee sports surgeons (and fellowships). We have an entire generation of orthopedists expertly knowledgeable in only *part* of the knee (sports surgery versus joint replacement surgery), not to mention orthopedists in general who have never had a specific interest in knees to begin with.

The LK-SS doctor

- Limited Knowledge: Not every orthopedist, rehabilitation doctor, or physical therapist is an expert on the knee!
- Suspect Scruples: For some doctors, it's all too tempting to recommend surgery.

Suspect Scruples: This is a delicate subject. As an orthopedist I am talking about my colleagues. These are people I work with, people I have helped train, people I see at every meeting, people I hope will come to my courses and buy my textbooks. But let's face it: a number of orthopedists and physiatrists are not walking the straight and narrow. They are a minority, but not a small one. Some of the less honest doctors are early in their practice and will do anything to get started in a competitive market; others are chairmen of departments

> who abuse their prestige. They work in small hospitals; they operate out of large university centers. They are friendly, smooth talking and persuasive. They work side by side with excellent, knowledgeable, trustworthy doctors from whom they are outwardly indistinguishable.

There are shades of dishonesty. Sometimes doctors are blatantly dishonest, such as when they state that a problem is in need of surgery, even when they know it isn't so. But there are more subtle forms of dishonesty: failing to correct a patient's misinformation and misunderstanding. For example, you might undergo a sophisticated test such as an MRI, the report of which will read "Grade 1 tear of the meniscus cartilage." You think, *torn cartilage! I need surgery*. Not so. A Grade 1 tear is invisible to the naked eye—if a tear at all—and requires no surgery; but the LK-SS surgeon will keep that information to him/herself and will happily allow you to sign the surgical consent form. To the LK-SS it's irresistible. What better scenario for a surgeon than a patient expecting surgery? The patient is unlikely to know that he or she would have done equally well with nonoperative measures.

Consider this next scenario: a person has a severe arthritic flare-up in their knee and consults a specialist. The pain is so bad that he or she will agree to anything—including surgery. Every orthopedist knows that the flare-up will quiet down, especially if this is the patient's first. But the LK-SS surgeon will gladly offer to eliminate the problem with a knee replacement—soon, before the pain wears off. Don't scoff. This scenario is not uncommon.

It is also deceitful to send the patient for physical therapy that is not tailored to the patient's specific condition. While some problems can improve with twenty minutes of heat packs and cycling on an exercise bicycle, many conditions require a more personal approach. But by sending you for plain, impersonal, bare-boned physical therapy that won't help you, the surgeon can tell your insurance carrier that you "failed physical therapy" and that you therefore need surgery.

Which brings us to the perfect crime: the surgeon picks a high-tech, outpatient procedure that is associated with a low complication rate and a speedy recovery. The procedure is performed on a patient who was going to do well anyway. When the patient gets better, the surgeon is credited with the recovery and is referred many more patients. Everybody wins—except the people paying the bills and the premium—but who cares?

Even educated people get tricked into surgery. I myself can imagine going to the dentist with a toothache and having the dentist send me for an expensive test. If the test came back saying I had some kind of dental rot, it wouldn't dawn on me to think that perhaps *every* test on *every* patient shows dental rot, and that my trusty dentist was using that test to sell me an unnecessary procedure. So I sympathize fully with people who've been sold a knee arthroscopy. Wherefore the existence of this book.

Physiatrists and chiropractors are not immune to the LK-SS phenomenon either: where surgeons exploit gullible patients by selling surgery, LK-SS physiatrists and chiropractors look for endless therapy sessions.

Interestingly, if this is a personal injury case, your attorney may play a role in your getting inappropriate advice and treatment, especially if he/she is an LK-SS attorney: when he sees cartilage tear, he will see this tear as the result of the injury (with a wink from the orthopedist). Of course, from a business point of view, he will not be displeased that you need surgery as it makes for a stronger legal case. Likewise, it makes for a stronger case if you are receiving ongoing physical therapy, as it demonstrates persistent symptoms and a need for prolonged care.

Faced with both a patient and (not infrequently) a lawyer who expect surgery and prolonged physical therapy, the LK-SS surgeon and physiatrist find it irresistible to schedule an operation and lengthy therapy.

In the following chapters we will review what you can do to protect yourself against misinformation and painfully suboptimal treatment.

CHAPTER 2
The Misleading MRI

Summary Soundbites:

- When it comes to knee pain, an MRI may or may not tell you what your real problem is.
- In the hands of the wrong orthopedist, the MRI becomes a license to operate.
- Doctors need to treat patients—not tests.

In the thirty or so years since its development, the MRI has gone from being a medical curiosity to a common source of misunderstanding. In fact, the accuracy of the MRI for meniscal tears is arguably one of the *greatest* sources of misunderstanding in the world of orthopedic surgery. Its roots lie in the awesome power of MRI technology.

What is an MRI?

MRI stands for Magnetic Resonance Imaging. It is an extraordinary tool that allows doctors to look inside the human body. It consists of a narrow flat table (or chair), on which the patient rests; patient and table are surrounded by a huge magnet. The MRI produces black-and-white pictures of the knee, shadows if you will. But as terrific as it is, the MRI creates nothing more than thin flat slices of a complex, colorful three-dimensional structure. Imagine trying to recreate in your mind the shape of a funny-looking loaf of bread just by observing the slices on a plate. MRIs are therefore subject to interpretation. Doctors with varying degrees of experience and knowledge will read MRIs differently.

Some of the conditions that may be missed on an MRI

- Early arthritis (Chapter 5)
- Pain coming down from the hip (Chapter 7)
- Kneecap malalignment (Chapter 6)
- Bruising of skin and nerves (Chapter 7)
- RSD (Chapter 7)
- A tight ilio-tibial band (Chapter 7)

MRIs are problematic in five ways:

1. MRIs can miss certain painful conditions:

    - <u>Arthritis.</u> Arthritis has a specific textbook definition: the loss of articular cartilage, the shiny white material at the end of each bone. Arthritis can be confined to a small part of the knee or can involve the entire knee. If the arthritic area is small enough, it will not be found on an MRI. This is a common source of patient disappointment. When patients go to an orthopedist complaining of knee pain, they are often told that they have torn cartilage; they expect that an outpatient operation will fix it; when the operation doesn't work, the doctor explains that he found some arthritis. "How could that be? It didn't say so on the MRI!" Caveat emptor! If you are over fifty years old and you have knee pain, you may well have an area of arthritis in your knee that will not show up on an MRI. A doctor should explain this to you before you embark on any arthroscopy.

- Ligament tears. Following a major injury, a completely shredded ligament will be detected on any MRI. However, an ACL which is partially torn—some of the fibers are normal, some are torn—may also appear normal on an MRI. This is because the traditional MRI slices are 4 mm thick. Everything within those 4 mm is averaged. Fortunately, a partially torn ligament can still function normally. I'll discuss this further in Chapter 4.
- Kneecap problems. The kneecap (patella) can be poorly aligned in many different ways. Most of the time, in my experience, the malalignment will be missed by the radiologist. In fact, a number of MRI centers do not even bother to take all the MRI cuts (views) necessary to judge the position of the kneecap. It saves money and few people complain. The kneecap can "ride high;" in other words it can sit too far from the knee joint. The medical term for this is patella alta. This is a condition people can be born with, in which case it is said to be congenital, and it can also be due to trauma. When the condition is traumatic, swelling and hemorrhage are present, and any radiologist can detect the abnormality. The congenital variety, however, is more subtle and many radiologists will miss it. There are other forms of malalignment that are likely to be overlooked on an MRI. This is a shame because kneecap pain is quite common and difficult to treat. When you are trying to convince the insurance companies that you have a real problem with your kneecap, it doesn't make life easier to be holding an MRI report erroneously read as normal (or simply "torn meniscus").
- Bruises of the skin and nerves. If you strike your knee and painfully bruise an underlying nerve, this will not be revealed on an MRI. This condition can be present in those who hit their knees against the dashboard of a car or fall onto their knees.

- Chondrocalcinosis. This is a biological condition whereby the soft tissues in your knee are filled with calcium crystals. Calcium is good for you when it's in your bone, not when it's in your cartilage. This can be a source of major pain. Ironically, though the condition shows up well on an x-ray, it may not show up at all on an MRI.

2. At the other extreme, MRIs can over-read select conditions:
    - Torn cartilage. The radiologist may feel that something is torn, and yet at surgery the structure is found to be intact. The reasons for this are complex and have to do with signal artifact. I need to backtrack a little and review with you what a meniscus looks like on an MRI. A perfectly normal meniscus on an ideal MRI picture appears as a solid black triangle, somewhat akin to a baseball pennant (Figure 2-1). Occasionally, one finds a blob of white or a tiny white line in the middle of the triangle. (Any variation from perfection on an MRI is called a signal change. It can be due to the MRI hardware or software, and it can also be introduced by scarring from prior surgery. Most commonly it merely reflects a biological variation within the meniscus (Figure 2-2).

        → One of the most questionable practices in radiology is the reporting of normal signal changes in meniscal cartilage as tears (Figure 2-2). In the early days of MR imaging, a grading system from I to III was devised. Grade I and II tears do not represent changes visible to the naked eye. Although some might argue that they represent tears at the microscopic level, they are not tears that one could see or would operate upon. (Some consider a Grade 2 tear to be a small tear; a nick so to speak.)

        → I was most shocked a few years ago when a radiologist showed me how he could simply dial in a Grade I or II tear by turning a knob on his MRI console!

        → This made it easier for me to understand how certain radiologists might read a tear on every MRI. By reporting

Grade I and II changes as tears, the radiologist allows the unscrupulous orthopedic surgeon to "sell" the patient a surgical procedure as most patients readily agree to surgery upon seeing the word tear.

→ In short, the MRI report has become a license to operate.

→ The insurers don't know any better and readily approve the procedure.

→ A Grade III change is more likely to represent a true tear (Figure 2-3). And even then, there can be false positives, the scientific term for false alarm. It is the doctor's responsibility to correlate the test results with the patient's symptoms and physical examination.

- Baker's cyst. In anticipation of a general outcry from my radiology colleagues, let me apologize ahead of time for including Baker's cysts in this section. Over one hundred years ago, Dr. Baker described a pouch of fluid commonly found at the back of the knee. The liquid is normal knee joint fluid that, in some people, seeps through a small opening and collects in this pouch. The pouch varies in size from person to person. It ranges from being invisible to feeling like a large ping-pong ball. The swelling can come and go as the fluid moves back and forth from the cyst to the knee joint. Unless the cyst is particularly large, it is usually asymptomatic and requires no treatment. According to current thinking, fluid tends to build up in the knee—thus filling up the Baker's cyst—when something is irritating the knee. That something can include any number of conditions including arthritis or a true torn meniscus. The situation is analogous to tears in your eye. If something were to irritate your eye, it would tear. (It is unfortunate that a tear of the meniscus and a tear in your eye are written the same way.) However, in the case of your eye, the tears escape down your cheek, whereas in the knee they have nowhere to go but into that Baker's cyst. The treatment of a Baker's cyst (which is rarely necessary) must therefore be focused on addressing the source of irritation within the knee (torn cartilage, arthritis, etc.).

- → To every rule there is an exception: occasionally, a one-way valve develops between the cyst and the knee: fluid can get into the cyst, but can't flow back to the joint. The body absorbs the fluid but not completely: it leaves behind a jelly-like substance that can actually harden with time. The doctor may place a needle in that cyst and aspirate (suck out) that substance. It may recur.
- → Most significantly, a Baker's cyst is readily seen on an MRI and it is commonly listed on the MRI report. Radiologists are perfectly justified in listing it (wherefore the above apology). The problem—and this is why I've listed the Baker's cyst in this section—is that everybody but the patient understands that it is a common, harmless finding. Patients are understandably anxious at the thought of a tumor-sounding cyst living around their knee. It is therefore not so much a question of an over-read by the radiologist as an over-interpretation on the part of the patient. It doesn't help that in the radiologist's summation, the innocent Baker's cyst is listed above the true culprit (arthritis, for example). See below.

- Bone tumors and infections. An MRI is so sensitive that it detects the smallest change in tissue composition. Such changes occasionally give the appearance of a tumor or an infection. This is quite frightening. Fortunately, a biopsy will reveal the tissue to be normal.

3. The MRI does not tell you what hurts.

It is common for people to have an abnormality which is completely asymptomatic (pain-free). The mere presence of an abnormality does not signify that there is a problem that must be treated, and it is the doctor who must decide whether the so-called abnormality is truly the source of the problem. I have seen countless patients who have had MRI abnormalities surgically corrected and who still complain of the same pain. For example, I once treated a patient with knee pain who had had surgery for a torn meniscus.

His MRI had clearly suggested a torn cartilage, but he still had pain despite the surgery. A further workup revealed that his knee pain was actually caused by a hip condition. The knee pain completely resolved once the hip was surgically repaired. This is by no means a rare scenario. The finding of a torn cartilage on an MRI is quite common, but does not automatically indicate the source of pain.

Some LK-SS orthopedists routinely dictate MRI-confirmed meniscal tear in their operative reports when describing the meniscus they have just "operated" on. If the surgery turns out to have been unwarranted, the surgeon can blame the MRI. "It's not my fault, Mrs. Jones, that I operated for nothing. That MRI report did report torn cartilage, did it not?"

4. MRI reports usually emphasize the wrong condition.

An MRI report commonly reads like this:

- tear of the meniscus
- water in the knee
- partial tear of such and such ligament
- Baker's cyst
- arthritis

While this report may technically be correct, the order of the conditions listed implies that the torn meniscus is the main problem. In most patients, however, the arthritis supersedes all other afflictions. The patient will not improve until the arthritis is addressed. Little tears of the meniscus, water in the knee, and partial tears of ligaments are not likely to be the source of the patient's pain. The bit about the tear of the meniscus *does* however succeed in catching the eye of the patient and the unsuspecting family doctor, and it paves the way for an offer from the orthopedist to fix that nasty little problem with a surgical procedure. (See sample MRI report at the end of this chapter.)

5. The Reverse Placebo Effect (see Chapter 9)

Patients given a diagnosis of a herniated disc, a torn rotator cuff, a torn ligament, a torn meniscus, a torn *anything* will think of themselves as wounded. This messes with their mind; they baby themselves; they can't do this; they can't do that. Of course, this protective behavior can on occasion be appropriate; but when the tear or herniation is but an MRI finding with no clinical relevance, the MRI report without appropriate counseling is harmful to the patient.

All MRIs are Not Equivalent

You would be appalled by the variations in image quality from one MRI to another and by the differences in accuracy from one report to another. This is a reflection of the diversity among the four elements that make up an MRI and its accompanying report: the hardware (the machine), the software (the computer program that runs the machine), the radiologist, and the orthopedist (the type of doctor most likely to be looking at your knee).

- The hardware: As with cars and planes, MRIs come in different models. The most obvious difference between them is their open versus closed nature. The closed models are tunnels into which a person is slid via a narrow table. The open models are open on the sides. By and large, the closed models are more precise. The main advantage of the open models lies in the diminished claustrophobia. Having said this, modern medications can dispel this claustrophobia, and a small Valium®-like tablet can nearly turn a closed MRI session into a relaxing experience. (Valium® itself is not used because it lasts too long.) Note: there now exist "extremity" MRIs. These are smaller MRIs for knees, feet, elbows, and hands. You sit and place your knee in the MRI. No sweat.

The variable ingredients of an MRI

- The machine.
- The computer software.
- The radiologist. He or she writes the report.
- The orthopedist. He or she reviews the MRI pictures and correlates them with your symptoms (or should).

The software: This runs the hardware, as it does in any computer, and it is as important as the machine itself. This explains why the most beautiful MRI images do not necessarily come from the very latest machines. Understandably, the information pertaining to the software and to the hardware is not something readily available to the lay or orthopedic public.

The radiologist: This person is vastly underestimated. The radiologist (and/or his technician) can manipulate the software to highlight certain features of the knee. Two radiologists using the same machine can obtain different results! The radiologist has to interpret (read) the pictures. Not all radiologists are equally adept at appreciating the subtleties of a knee MRI. What looks essentially normal to one radiologist can look somewhat irregular, swollen, displaced, or degenerated to another. What one radiologist reads as a tear, another reads as a simple signal change (radiology jargon for a white or black spot on a magnetic image).

Don't be fooled by the term Board Certified under a radiologist's name. Board certification doesn't make him or her an expert in every area of radiology. I am Board Certified in Orthopedic Surgery, but you wouldn't want me as the main surgeon on your spine!

Remember also: by and large, no radiologist can tell you what hurts. A radiologist has not taken a medical history from you and hasn't examined you.

The orthopedist: This is the person who should be correlating the MRI images with your symptoms. Some doctors simply read the radiologist's report and read you the alleged diagnosis. This is a major mistake for the reasons listed above.

Note that the best orthopedist and the best radiologist can still disagree on whether there is a cartilage or ligament tear or not, and they can disagree on whether the kneecap is normal or not. You would think that a radiologist would be more knowledgeable than an orthopedist when it comes to reading x-rays and MRIs, and sometimes this is true. But, in certain cases, it is the reverse.

The buck stops with the clinician looking after you. If an MRI is necessary to make the diagnosis, he (or she) must review the films himself.

The MRI-Confirmed Tear

It is not uncommon to find this term in doctors' notes or legal documents. A typical sentence would read, "Ms. Smith sustained an MRI-confirmed tear of the medial meniscus." By now you understand the problem. With the possible exception of grade 3 tears, the MRI hasn't confirmed anything. And yet, in a "see no evil, hear no evil, speak no evil" mode, surgeons looking to perform an arthroscopy or attorneys looking for dollars will gladly lean on the MRI report for support.

The LIPs of the World. The lawyers, insurance companies, and patients collectively and individually represent very powerful groups. As of this writing, licensed independent practitioners (LIPs) tend to assume that MRIs are perfect. They assume that anything that is wrong will show up on an MRI; they rely on the MRI report as if it came from a higher power, and they readily accept the concept that any abnormality on the MRI is painful and needs to be fixed. As we have seen above, nothing could be further from the truth. This attitude, however, plays directly into the hands of LK-SS orthopedists, and it completely skewers insurance and legal payouts. Patients with painful conditions that are not apparent to the radiologist are denied coverage and compensation, while people with fictitious tears can be given significant rewards.

A misleading MRI report in multiple respects. (See also subsequent chapters.)

Imprecise Radiology Associates
425 Main Street
Anywhere, USA

Aymnot Thorough, MD
13 Dontno Avenue
Mainstream, USA
Re: Mr. UR Snookered

MRI of the Right Knee

An MRI of the knee in the axial, sagittal, and coronal images was performed.

A joint effusion is noted. There is a tear of the posterior horn of the medial meniscus. The lateral meniscus is within normal limits. There is a partial tear of the medial collateral ligament and of the anterior cruciate ligament. Severe chondromalacia with subchondral sclerosis can be found in the medial femoral condyle. The remainder of the study is unremarkable.

IMPRESSION:
Joint effusion
Tear of the posterior horn of the medial meniscus
Partials tears of the medial collateral and anterior cruciate ligaments
Severe chondromalacia of the medial compartment.

____

BS, MD
Board Certified Radiologist

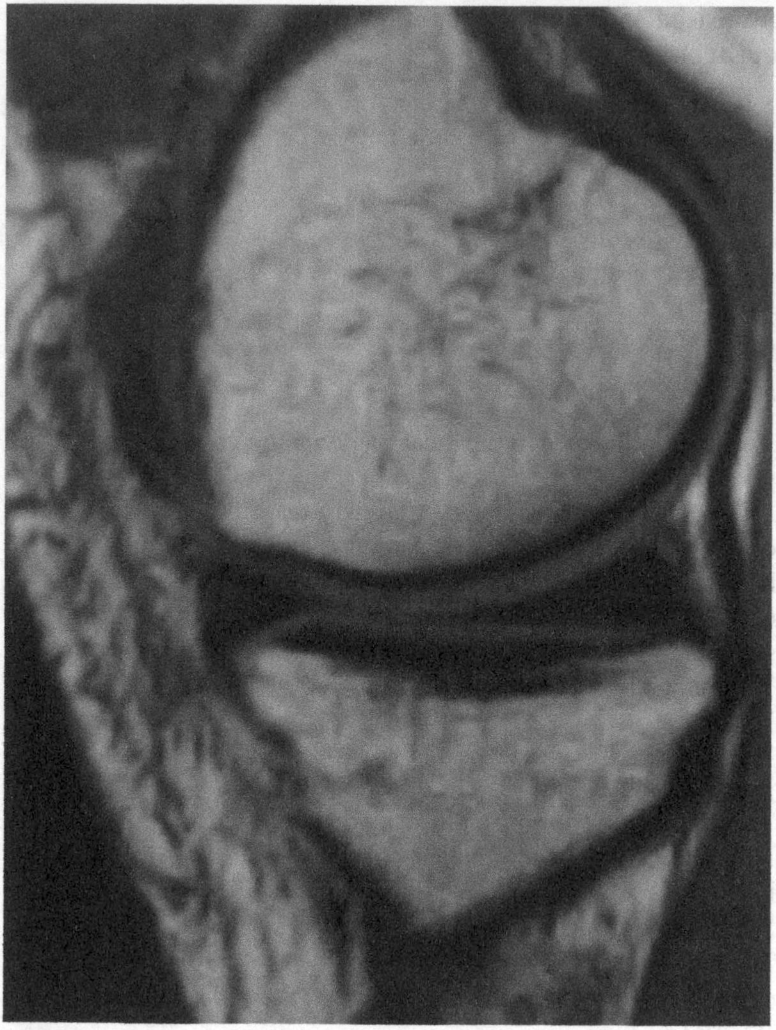

Figure 2-1. Side view of a normal meniscus. The front and back portions (the "horns") appear as solid black triangles. (If you look with a magnifying glass, you might see a bit of white within those triangles. This might be labeled by some as a Grade 1 tear. It's not a tear in any common sense of the word.

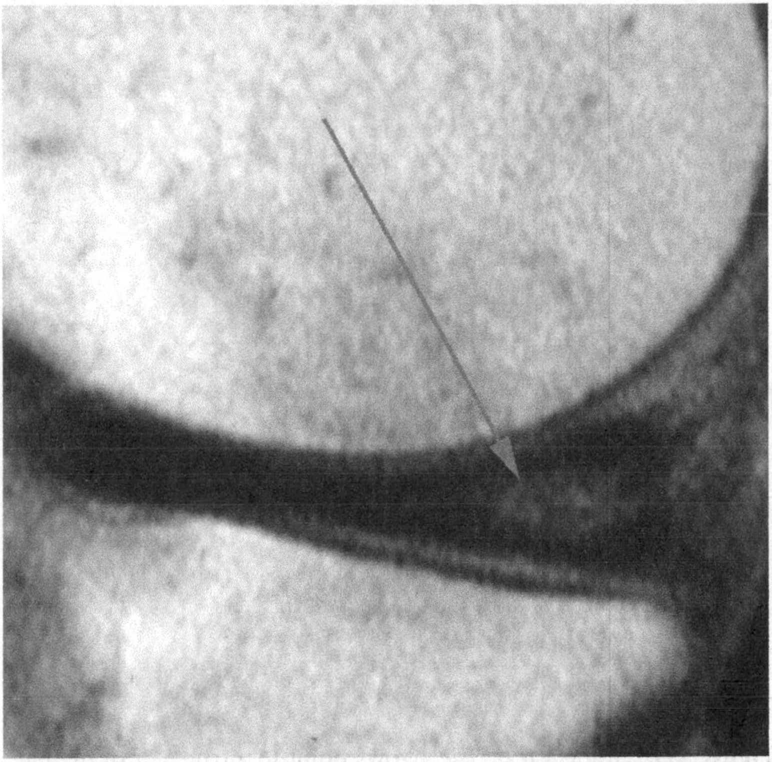

Figure 2-2. Grade 2 tear: The white signal within the meniscus represents a biochemical change within the meniscus not visible (or barely visible) to the naked eye.

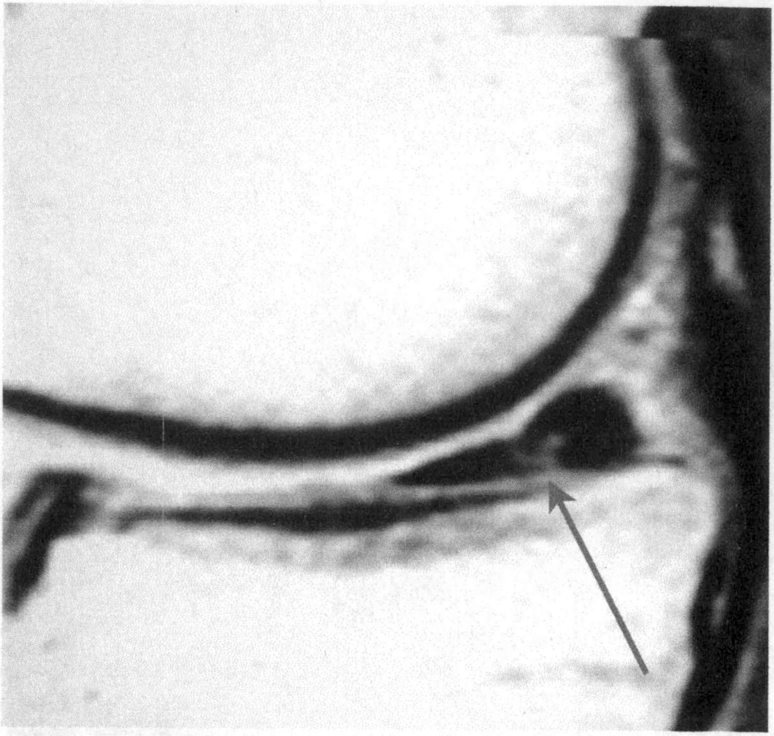

Figure 2-3. Grade 3 tear. The arrows point to a true tear of the meniscus. The meniscus appears to be in two pieces, and this would be visible to the naked eye. Such a tear can potentially be painful.

CHAPTER 3

Life-Threatening Torn Cartilage

"Blake Griffin will have minor surgery on his right knee this week… The [team] said the surgery would be a "routine arthroscopic procedure." *New York Times*, December 20 2016.

There's no minor surgery, only minor surgeons.

Summary Soundbites:

- At the dawn of this new millennium, you are at greater risk of being misdiagnosed with a torn cartilage than at any other time in history.
- Nearly every MRI report reads "torn meniscus."
- Not every meniscal tear hurts.
- Most tears do not require surgery.

<u>Bad news:</u> there's a good chance that an MRI will show that you have torn cartilage in your knee.
<u>More bad news:</u> if this report lands in the hands of an LK-SS orthopedist[1] you will be told that you need surgery.
<u>Good news:</u> he's pulling your leg. Chances are that you don't need surgery.

Once upon a time, surgery for a torn cartilage required one or two big incisions about the knee. Surgeons thought twice about performing this kind of surgery. No more.

[1] Limited Knowledge - Suspect Scruples (see Chapter 1).

Now that the procedure is "minor," unscrupulous surgeons perform these at a remarkable clip.

Cartilage is both:

- o The shiny white material at the end of a bone.
- o The rubbery shock absorbers inside the knee.

What is a Torn Cartilage?

Cartilage. The medical profession is responsible for having coined one term for two very different structures: Cartilage is the name given to the smooth white material which lines the end of bones—check it out the next time you eat chicken. This cartilage is never torn, but it may wear out. The wearing out process is called arthritis.

Cartilage is also the colloquial name given to the thin rubbery shock absorbers inside the knee between the thighbone (femur) and shinbone (tibia) known in the medical world as the menisci (pronounced "men-IS-kai:" one meniscus, two menisci). (Figure 3-1). These structures can be torn, wherefore the term torn cartilage.

Menisci are crescent-shaped and there are two in each knee—one toward the inner part of the knee (medial) and the other toward the outside (lateral). By virtue of their somewhat crescent/cupped shape they add stability to the knee. In other words, they help keep the knees from being wobbly. Because of their cushy nature, they also provide shock absorption.

When the doctor says, "You have torn cartilage" he is referring to one (or both) of those menisci.

How does a cartilage tear?

1. A sudden injury. You get tackled, you feel a pop, and can't straighten the knee. Chances are you tore a meniscus.
2. Wear and tear. Most tears fall into this category. The natural aging process causes chemical changes in the meniscus, more so in some people than in others. These changes in turn

predispose the meniscus to fraying and tearing much as might an old carpet. The posterior (toward the back of the knee) aspect of the meniscus is subject to higher stresses than the rest of the meniscus, and research suggests that the back of the meniscus is also mechanically weaker. Not surprisingly then, it is the most likely part of the meniscus to tear. Although a specific event may bring the tear to light, the tear has often been there all along.

What does a torn cartilage feel like?

It doesn't necessarily hurt; but if it's painful, the pain is usually localized to one specific part of the knee. You can just about put your finger on it. With the knee bent at a right angle, as when sitting in a chair, the tenderness is typically right between the thighbone and the shinbone, the so-called joint line. Bending down is particularly painful. When there is a large "bucket handle" tear (see below), you can't completely straighten out the knee. (Keep in mind that even minor ligament injuries can also cause this for a few days after the trauma. See Chapter 4).

What other conditions feel like a torn cartilage?

There are many causes of knee pain. If you are between the ages of twenty and forty you may simply have a nagging tendinitis, that is, an inflammation of a tendon; you may have a subtle problem with your kneecap (Chapter 6); you could be suffering from runner's knee, an irritation of the so-called iliotibial band running along the outside of the leg and knee (Chapter 7).

The MRI report may indicate torn cartilage, but the *real* cause of your pain may be one of the conditions listed above. As noted repeatedly in this book, many people without knee pain can appear to have a torn cartilage on an MRI. Therefore the mere presence of such a torn cartilage does *not* indicate the source of a person's pain.

What does a torn cartilage look like?

A meniscus can tear in an infinite variety of ways: there are so-called bucket handle, parrot-beak, radial, cleavage, flap, and degenerative tears—and every permutation thereof (Figures 3-2 and 3-3). A bucket-handle tear is usually large and involves a major portion of the meniscus. The other forms of meniscal tears are usually localized to the back of the meniscus. The back and front portions of the meniscus are called "horns." Therefore a common finding on an MRI report is "a tear of the posterior horn of the medial meniscus."

Are all tears equivalent?

No. Radiologists have graded tears into categories I, II, and III (See Chapter 2). Grade I tears represent chemical changes or scratches not visible to the naked eye. A grade III tear represents a through-and-through tear that is clearly visible (Figure 3-3).

This is a critical difference.

A Grade III tear may or may not require surgery. A Grade I tear does not! Every orthopedic surgeon knows this. The LK-SS surgeon, however, routinely counts on your ignorance to sell you an operation for a Grade I tear. (The term "Grade 2" varies among radiologists.)

Can I get arthritis from a torn cartilage?

This is a common scare tactic to get you to surgery. "Let's take care of this before you get arthritis." Nonsense medicine is what this is. In the first place, the common little tears that you find on MRI reports will not cause arthritis: as you understand by now, most torn cartilages found on MRI reports have little connection to reality. By and large, true tears occur in older patients and are of the degenerative (i.e. wear-and-tear) type. They are equivalent to a worn carpet. They may be associated with arthritis but do not *cause* arthritis.

On the other hand, large sudden tears of the meniscus do present a potential problem. In addition to causing pain, the torn piece can in certain cases rub against the articular cartilage, wear it down and theoretically cause arthritis (see Chapter 5).

Until thirty years ago, surgeons would remove an entire meniscus to treat a meniscal tear. The meniscus was felt to be a useless structure, the appendix of the knee so to speak. We now know better. Removing the entire meniscus greatly increases a person's risk of arthritis. This is presumably because the knee's shock absorber has been removed and the knee has been rendered somewhat less stable. (We do not know how much meniscus has to be removed to significantly increase someone's risk for arthritis.) Nowadays, surgeons therefore remove as little meniscus as possible—the torn portion, no more no less. A partial meniscectomy is performed.

The younger the patient, the less the surgeon removes: if arthritis develops in an older patient, there is always the option of a knee replacement. That option is not as palatable to the younger patient (see Chapter 5). In fact, there is *no* great option when treating arthritis in the younger patient. The best treatment is therefore prevention, and prevention in this case means leaving as much of the meniscus as possible.

Do even educated people get tricked into surgery?

You bet. As noted in Chapter 1, educated or not you tend to trust your doctor.

The Physical Examination

In the days before MRIs, your doctor would make the diagnosis of a torn meniscus by listening to your story (the history) and by examining your knee. You can still make a strong case for the following point of view: a significant tear of the meniscus is best diagnosed on the physical examination.

If the tear is very large as in, say, a bucket-handle tear (see Figure 3-2), the torn piece will interfere with the mechanics of the knee. The knee will lock up. It's as if you dropped a stone in a big machine. The knee won't straighten or will refuse to bend. You will feel a mechanical stop. The knee will bend and straighten freely until it reaches a certain point. It will then seem to be blocked as if by a doorstop. The doctor then has his first clue. Mind you, it takes a very big tear to cause such locking. Conversely, there is hardly anything else that can cause such predictable and reproducible locking. You could argue convincingly that an MRI is unnecessary in this setting.

The meniscus lives between the thighbone and shinbone in a space that is easy to palpate when the knee is bent. This space is called "the joint space." When a meniscus is torn, the tissues around it become inflamed. An analogy can be made here with a hangnail. In fact, in many ways, a torn meniscus *is* a hangnail of the knee. The inflammation around the torn meniscus causes pain, and when the doctor presses his finger against the joint space it hurts! This finding is present with just about any significant tear. It is also found in the presence of arthritis and is therefore not specific for a meniscal tear. Nevertheless, it provides yet another clue for the doctor. In a patient not likely to have arthritis, namely someone under forty, it is an even bigger clue.

A classic test for a torn meniscus is the McMurray test. The patient lies on his or her back. The knee is bent all the way back. The doctor straightens the knee while turning the foot. If a dull clunk is perceived, the test is considered positive for a torn meniscus. Alas, this test is too inaccurate: you can have a painfully torn meniscus without having a positive McMurray test, and a positive McMurray test does not automatically indicate the presence of a significant tear. The following story illustrates the point. Frank Stinchfield, MD, at one time the preeminent orthopedist in the United States and the teller of this story, went to visit Dr. McMurray in Great Britain. Dr. McMurray had just published his "McMurray test" and was eager to demonstrate it.

"Lie down Frank," he said, "and I'll show you how it's done."

Dr. Stinchfield hiked himself up onto the examination table and bared his knee. McMurray performed his test and they both heard a dull pop. "Why Frank, you have a torn meniscus!"

"Amazing," replied Dr. Stinchfield, "my knee doesn't even hurt. Let me try it on you."

With that he traded places with McMurray and performed the test. They both heard a clunk. "Wow," said Dr. Stinchfield, "you have a tear too!"

"Nonsense," snapped McMurray, "let's go for lunch."

So much for the McMurray test.

Nevertheless doctors will note "positive McMurray test" in their office notes to impress upon the insurance company the need for a surgical procedure.

Another test is the Apley grind. Here the patient lies on his or her stomach with the knee bent at a right angle. The doctor pushes on the heel and twists the leg as if to grind the knee into the examination table. The idea is to perform a little watusi on the torn meniscus and elicit pain. The problem here is that unless the patient is quite small and slender, it is difficult for the doctor to simulate with his arm the forces generated by the patient when he or she carries out the normal activities of daily living. As with the McMurray, a positive Apley means little: just about any knee condition can hurt with the Apley maneuver.

Do you need surgery for a torn cartilage?

Yes, you do need surgery if your knee pain is clearly the result of a tear and the pain interferes significantly with your everyday activities. Believe it or not, it is not always easy to determine at first glance whether torn cartilage is or is not the source of your pain.

First of all, the torn cartilage seen on the MRI may not be a tear at all. Little changes that are of no consequence are routinely read as cartilage tears (see above and Chapter 2).

What's worse, these little changes can be introduced by the radiologist simply by the turn of a dial. These so-called false-positive tears are the knee equivalent of a false alarm.

In my experience, the odds of coming across a false-positive MRI range from 10 percent to 100 percent depending on the knowledge and integrity of the radiologist. Since a reading of torn meniscus presents the unscrupulous orthopedist with a license to operate, an equally unscrupulous radiologist reads a torn meniscus in essentially everyone. This insures him continued business from the orthopedist and/or lawyer.

Secondly, not all tears are painful. The knowledgeable orthopedist will carefully examine other parts of the knee before pronouncing the meniscus the likely source of pain. The LK-SS, alas, will pounce on the MRI report and announce that he has found the source of your pain without ever looking for the other causes.

A torn cartilage can be problematic because it is painful or because it causes locking. *Locking* is the term used when the knee won't straighten because something is blocking it. That something is the piece of cartilage interfering with the intricate machinery of the knee. Again, the consumer must beware: there is so-called pseudo-locking whereby a knee won't straighten or bend simply because it hurts too much to do so. The knowledgeable orthopedists can tell the difference. The LK-SS will use the pseudo-locking to, once again, sell an operation. "Mrs. Smith, your knee is locked. We better get to this quickly."

No, you do not need surgery unless your knee pain is most likely the result of the tear and the pain interferes significantly with your activities of daily living.

If You Do Need Surgery

Is surgery an emergency?

NEVER. There is no such thing as life-threatening torn cartilage.

The LK-SS surgeon takes the shoe-salesman approach (no offense meant to shoe salesmen): make the sale today—or lose the customer. This may be reasonable in the retail world; it is downright unethical in the setting of a possible torn cartilage. Unless the knee is locked, cartilage surgery can always wait—and even then, it need not be done that day. Don't let yourself get pressured into signing on the dotted line.

The "miracle" of microsurgery and laser surgery

In keeping with the tone of this book, I am pulling your leg a little: there is no microsurgery for torn cartilage and there is no miracle of laser surgery, electrofrequencywhooziewhatsie, or anything else you can't pronounce.

These terms, however, are commonly used by doctors to dazzle you and to liposuck the common sense out of your head. Microsurgery has a very specific meaning in the world of surgery: surgery performed with the use of an operating room microscope. When severed tendons, ligaments, and blood vessels are reattached, the surgeon not uncommonly resorts to microsurgery.

No microscope is used in meniscus surgery, and therefore there is no microsurgery.

Lasers: The term laser is an acronym for light amplification by stimulated emission of radiation, not, as some cynics would have it, limited applications of sophisticated and expensive research. In conventional arthroscopic surgery, the orthopedist employs small instruments to snip at torn tissue. When using a laser instead, the surgeon heats the tissue until it is vaporized. The end result is the same. I myself operated with an advanced holmium laser for six months and taught laser safety for a major medical laser manufacturer; so, if anything, I am partial to lasers and related devices. Having said this, the advantage of a laser in the setting of a torn cartilage is essentially nonexistent. A laser does not speed up the surgery, does not improve recovery, and does not diminish the risks of surgery. If a surgeon tries to impress you with the use of a laser (or *any* related device), you know you are dealing with an

LK-SS. As of this writing, lasers in knee surgery are mainly used as a marketing tool. Many patients are impressed at the thought of having a laser procedure or microsurgery. Doctors and hospitals know this.

The true miracle

Because meniscus surgery is performed so frequently, it is easy to lose sight of the fact that it does represent a small miracle of technology. The procedure used to address torn cartilage is called an *arthroscopy* (ar-THROS-cup-ee) from the Greek "arthro" (joint) and "scop" (to look). A slender pencil-like tube is introduced into the knee. The tube is connected to a palm-sized camera which itself is connected to a television monitor. Thus, the inside of your knee is projected onto the television screen.

Note that nowhere in the word "arthroscopy" does the word "knee" appear. Indeed an arthroscopy can be performed on any joint, and a scope can be performed in any body cavity: cystoscopy (bladder), fundoscopy (uterus), and laparoscopy (abdomen) to name but a few.

Through a separate puncture hole, smallish instruments are introduced. These instruments are long, slender rods connected to miniaturized scissors, clippers, and shavers. They come in a multitude of shapes designed to reach the various nooks and crannies inside the knee; due to magnification they appear quite large on arthroscopy pictures, but they are in fact small (Figure 3-4).

Although most patients do not want to hear or see anything, it is possible for the person undergoing the procedure to observe the surgery on the same TV screen that is being watched by the surgeon (you may not be allowed to wear your glasses or contact lenses!).

One chooses between four anesthetics:

1. General anesthesia (intubation) whereby you are put to sleep via an intravenous medication and your respiration is assured via a plastic tube gently slipped down your windpipe. With just the

right amount of intravenous medication, it is possible to wake up rather quickly and be on your way home in just a few hours.

2. A spinal. A local anesthetic is injected in your lower back. This is below your spinal cord, and as such, paralysis is not a realistic complication. With this approach, you can remain wide-awake if you so desire or you can receive intravenous sedation which knocks you out, though not as deeply as with general anesthesia. It may take a few hours for the spinal to wear off, and in the meantime you must stay in the recovery room.
3. Local anesthetic. A Novocain-type of medication is injected directly into the knee. In my experience, this is the least reliable type of anesthesia. Because there are many folds and crevices in the knee, the medication may not reach each and every spot. The person opting for this has to be willing to accept the possibility of some pain and has to understand that they may require intravenous sedation. How long one stays in the recovery room after a local depends strictly on how much added sedation was given during the surgery.
4. A variation of general anesthesia is the use of a rubber diaphragm, or LMA (laryngeal mask airway), placed in the back of the throat. This is essentially general anesthesia without a tube down the windpipe. Depending on which anesthesiologist you speak to, this technique combines either the best or the worst of both worlds. I have had good success with this on my patients.

In my experience, these options are all approximately equal except for the local anesthetic for the reasons listed above. If the anesthesiologist has a strong preference for one approach or the other, I tend to go with that approach. The anesthesiologist is one person I hate to upset.

What is Band-Aid® surgery?

Band-Aid® surgery is the same as "minor surgery": surgery on somebody else. The terms Band-Aid® surgery and minor surgery are used to impress upon you that the procedure will be quick, painless, and risk-free. You won't need a surgical dressing, just a Band-Aid®. This is *relatively* true. The procedure itself is quick, but there can be a day and a half of pain thereafter. The chance of getting a significant complication is low but not zero. Infections, though rare, can occur. They lead to a significant amount of pain, further surgery, and a long course of antibiotics that may need to be administered intravenously. Some patients develop severe stiffness, and yet others develop a painful condition called Reflex Sympathetic Dystrophy (RSD) whereby pain fibers refuse to shut down and continue to send painful signals to the brain (see Chapter 7). As for just using a Band-Aid®, some people can get a fair amount of oozing for a day or so after surgery, and it is simply not appropriate to place such a small bandage.

When can I get my leg wet after surgery?

Within a few days, the puncture holes are reasonably sealed. Therefore, as soon as the dressing is off, I allow patients to shower. Water might still theoretically seep in if the leg were *soaked* in water, and because of this, I do not allow bathing or swimming until ten days or so after surgery. There are differences of opinion on this.

Recovery and Rehabilitation

Do you need physical therapy? When do you go back to work?

The beauty of performing surgery through two or three small puncture holes is that the recovery is infinitely faster than surgery carried out through a long skin incision. If you can be driven to work and if your work is sedentary, you can be back at work in one to two days. If you take a bus or subway or if you must stand on your feet a great deal, ten days is a more reasonable time to take off. Keep in mind that everyone is different. Resist the temptation to compare yourself to someone else. In some cases the knee has to be gently twisted during surgery for the surgeon to gain access to the torn cartilage, and this can prolong the recovery.

I find that approximately 50 percent of patients need physical therapy. People who within a few days of surgery still have trouble straightening the knee or bending it to 90 degrees are good candidates for formal physical therapy. Patients who find their leg to be wobbly and are not good at exercising on their own are also sent for physical therapy. Contrary to what we find with kneecap problems, therapy following arthroscopic cartilage surgery is reasonably standard from facility to facility: the therapist will apply heat and gently work on moving the knee. So-called modalities such as ultrasound can also be soothing. The therapist will stretch and massage the structures around the knee that have tightened up.

Can I exercise on my own after surgery?

If you have the discipline, the answer is absolutely yes. You may want one session of physical therapy to verify that you are performing the exercises correctly, but then you can certainly be on your own.

First, you want to make sure that your knee straightens all the way. (A painful knee wants to stay slightly bent.) Sit on the floor or a firm mattress with the leg out straight and work on getting the back of the knee up against that surface. Hold the muscles tight for about ten seconds. Count to three and start again. Do this for five to ten minutes at a time. It will seem like an eternity. I recommend music or television to fight the boredom.

At the opposite extreme, you want the knee to bend. The knee will be puffy from the fluid that was pumped through during the surgery, but you should be able to flex to 90 degrees (a right angle) within a few days. Sit on a table or bar stool, support your leg with the top of the other foot, and gradually let the knee bend.

It's amazing how quickly muscles become weak. Both fluid in the knee and pain can lead to muscle atrophy in the blink of an eye. Fortunately, this is easily reversible. Once you've regained reasonable motion in the knee—straightening it all the way and bending it 90 degrees—you can begin to strengthen it.

Start with the classic straight leg raise. Lie down, and without bending the knee, lift the heel an inch or so off the ground. Hold it off the ground about ten seconds. Count to three and repeat. Continue five to ten minutes at a time. It's as boring as it is effective (see above). When this becomes too easy, attach a light weight to the ankle (one pound) and repeat. The lower leg acts as a long lever arm, so one pound at the ankle is more impressive than it sounds, especially on a painful knee. You can then progress in one- to two-pound increments. You'll know when you're pretty much back to where you were before surgery.

Leg extensions. This is another classic exercise whereby you sit on a table or bar stool, and gradually straighten the knee. I recommend starting with a one-pound weight at the ankle and then *gradually* working up to heavier weights. Again, remember: the lower leg is a long lever. The effect of the weight on your ankle gets multiplied by the length of this lever. Go easy on weight increases. One- to two-pound increases are reasonable.

Are there exercises to avoid? Absolutely: wall slides are one example. For this exercise, you place your back flush against the wall and gradually assume a sitting position. The further away your feet are from the wall, the harder it is. It's a fine exercise for people with good knees looking to get stronger legs. It puts terrific stress on your kneecap though, and for many people this is painful. Try it if you want, but don't insist if it's the least bit painful.

"No pain, no gain"? This is a common adage. When a joint is stiff, it is reasonable to expect some discomfort as it is being stretched. But *no* strengthening exercise should be painful. If it is, back off on the weights or stop altogether.

Is pool therapy recommended?

Absolutely. People with pools barely need physical therapy in this setting. Being buoyant makes it easier to stand on the leg. Moving the leg in the water provides natural resistance. Kicking in the water (any style) is a solid strengthening exercise (ever see swimmers' legs?). Lakes work well too, although water that is too cold can make you tense up. I do not care for oceans if there are any waves or if there are sudden drop-offs. This is too dangerous. You need a warm, controlled environment. (Try a trip to the Caribbean. Medicare and insurances routinely cover that.)

Moist heat or dry heat?

Even though they are opposites, heat and cold can both be soothing. For straightforward exercises, the traditional approach is to "warm up, ice down." Massage the knee and apply heat, in any form, prior to exercise. Five minutes should be fine. At the end of the exercise apply a cold pack. If you are looking to control pain, I would alternate heat and cold every five to ten minutes until you find which is best for you. I would then use whichever you've chosen for as much of the day as is practical for you.

Trick of the trade: Rather than hold the heat or cold pack in your hands, wrap an elastic bandage (e.g., Ace®) once or twice around the knee. Then apply the cold/heat pack. Finish wrapping the bandage; the heat/cold pack stays in place. There are also commercially available neoprene wraps that will do this for you in an even more convenient manner.

Heat can be dry as when a heating pad is used or moist when a hot towel or electric hydrocollator is used. From a medical point of view, both are acceptable. You should use the form that works best for you.

Unusual Conditions

A small percentage of the population walks around with a so-called "discoid meniscus." This is a meniscus that looks like a poker chip rather than a crescent. Discoid menisci come in different flavors: an *incomplete* discoid meniscus has an opening in the middle.

The opening can be small or large. An incomplete discoid meniscus therefore can come close to looking like a normal meniscus, or at the other extreme, can essentially look like the traditional, complete discoid variety. The discoid meniscus can have normal peripheral attachments to the knee or can be completely detached from the back of the knee (the Wrisberg type of discoid meniscus). A Wrisberg discoid meniscus can cause snapping which eventually becomes painful. Surgery is required. It is challenging surgery because the meniscus has *never* been normally attached to the knee. There are no natural connections between the discoid meniscus and the knee capsule, and in fact, the meniscus can be quite a distance from where it should be. This is very different from a *normal* meniscus that becomes detached and which needs to be *re*-attached.

The treatment of a discoid meniscus consists of removing part of the meniscus (a partial meniscectomy). As usual, the surgeon will try to remove as little as possible for fear of predisposing his patient to early arthritis. On the other hand, because the meniscus can be so abnormal, it may require nearly total removal before the patient becomes asymptomatic (pain free). One has to hope that by the time our young patients develop arthritis we will have even more treatment options than we have today.

How to interpret your operative arthroscopy report

"Whoa, that's scary" is how you might react upon seeing your knee arthroscopy report.

Indeed, your surgeon may have alleged that he found tears of both menisci; loose bodies; a torn anterior cruciate ligament; articular cartilage lesions; arthritis; synovitis—or any combination thereof. Accordingly, he may state that he performed a "medial and lateral meniscectomy," a removal of loose bodies "through a separate incision," electrothermal shrinkage of your ACL, an "abrasion arthroplasty," and a multicompartment synovectomy.

Sometimes all of this is true. Usually it is only partially true. Occasionally none of it is true.

To grasp how this would be possible you need to understand how surgeons bill for arthroscopies: à la carte. By and large, the more they find wrong, the more things they can say were fixed, and the more they can bill. I was once asked to review a case where an orthopedist charged $45,000 for a twenty-minute routine arthroscopy. He'd "only" been paid $12,000 and was appealing to get more.

Take the case of the torn meniscus: you could have **a**) a significant pain-producing tear; **b**) a small tear akin to a little cuticle on your finger tip and of no significance; **c**) no tear at all.

In the first case, a surgeon is completely justified in billing for a "meniscectomy" whereby the offending torn meniscal portion is removed.

In the second case, the surgery (and billing) aren't warranted, but the surgeon will say, "I never said how big the tear was, and I have the right to have trimmed it and billed for it." This would be ethically very questionable.

The third case is outright insurance fraud.

How about the ACL ligament tear (see Chapter 4)? Some orthopedists will touch the ligament with a hot probe and bill for a full reconstruction. There are a number of problems with this: the concept of "shrinking" the stretched ACL fibers has long been discredited. Secondly, billing for a major reconstruction when all you've done is touch the ligament with a probe, well, need I say more? This is such low-lying fruit that some orthopedists at the bottom of the ethics chain can't help but find a stretched ACL even in a knee without the slightest *reason* for a tear and without the slightest *evidence* for a tear on the MRI.

A surgeon doesn't necessarily get paid to remove a small loose body (a free-floating pebble made of bone and/or cartilage). However, if the loose body is so large that the surgeon has to make a separate incision *or* if the loose body is larger than 5 mm, that can tip the scale in favor of the surgeon being paid. This might explain the 7 mm loose body that did not appear on the MRI or the separate incision that you just can't find on your skin. (I apologize for the cynicism, but some of this you just can't make up.)

If your articular cartilage is unhealthy (see Chapter 5), the surgeon may choose to freshen it up by shaving it. This is akin to mowing the lawn. This would be a débridement and the surgeon can bill for that (even though the benefit of this procedure is debatable). If there is *no* cartilage left over a well-defined area, the surgeon can roughen up the bone with a burr in an attempt to stimulate new cartilage formation. This is an "abrasion." A surgeon gets paid more for an abrasion than for a simple debridement, so . . . don't be completely surprised to find an abrasion in your operative report. (Let me emphasize that in your particular case the abrasion may indeed have been performed and may have been perfectly appropriate.)

Synovium is the cotton candy–like material found in various amounts within the knee. When it is more abundant than usual or when it is red and inflamed, one has "synovitis." Of course, the "more abundant than usual" is completely in the eye of the surgeon. The surgeon may get paid for performing a synovectomy whereby he/she removes excess synovium, and the payment is even greater if the synovectomy is performed in more than one compartment of the knee. So if the surgeon finds absolutely nothing wrong (and refuses to make up any of the conditions listed above) there can always be . . . synovitis.

"How can all of this be allowed?" you ask. I've been asking myself that question too. Since 1985.

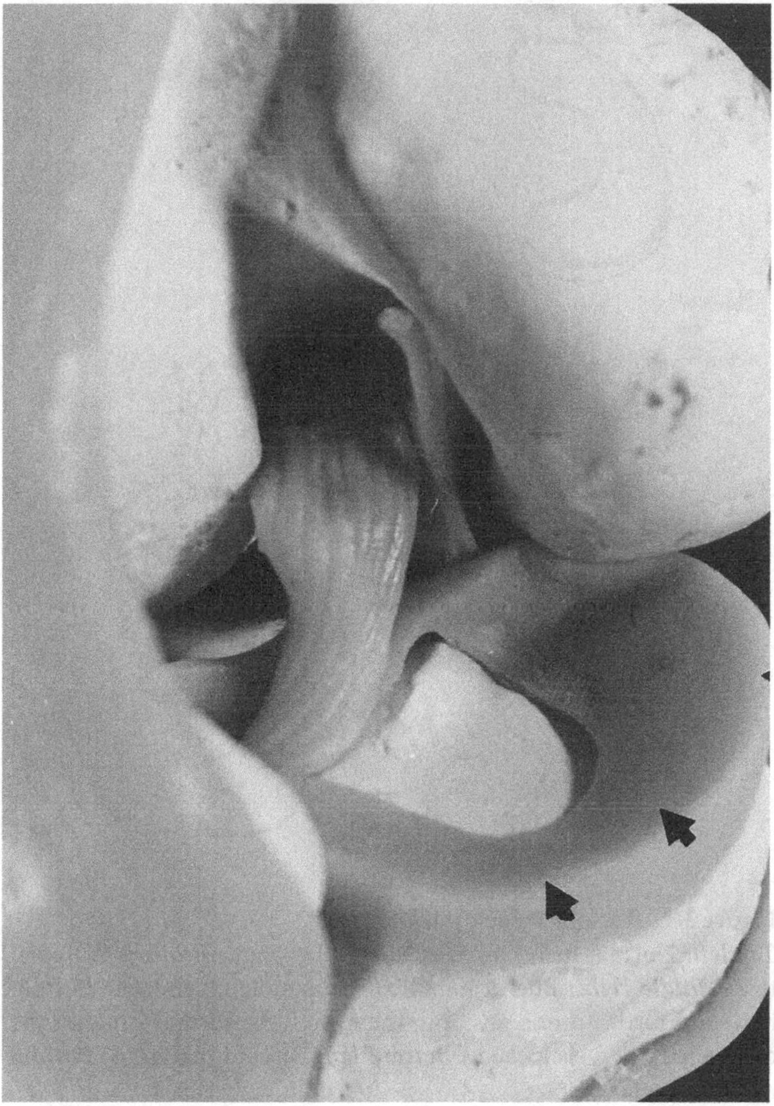

Figure 3-1. Model of a right knee. The arrows point to the medial (inner) meniscus.

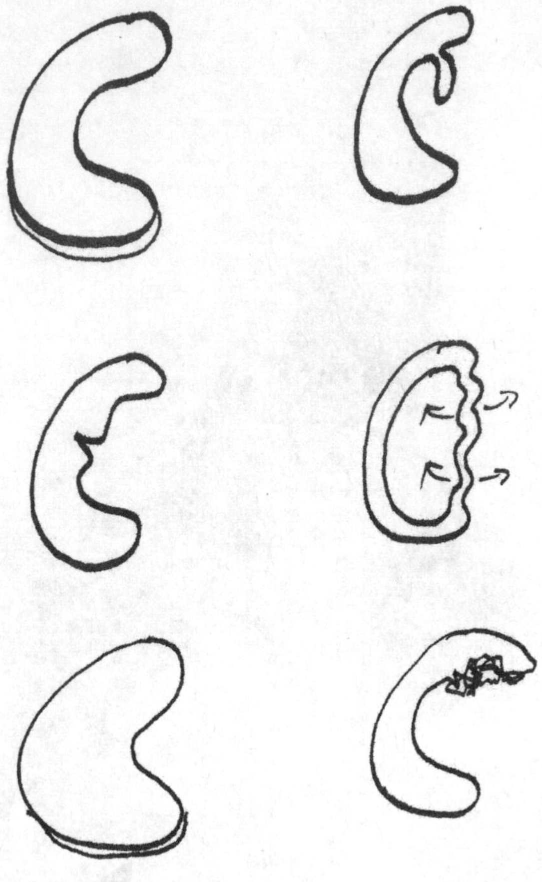

Figure 3-2. Various meniscal tears
Top left: Normal meniscus. ***Top right:*** Flap tear. ***Middle left:*** Radial tear. ***Middle right:*** Bucket handle. (The 'handle' of the tear can flip back and forth. In one position, the knee feels normal while in the other the knee feels locked.) ***Bottom left:*** Discoid meniscus. ***Bottom right:*** Complex tear.

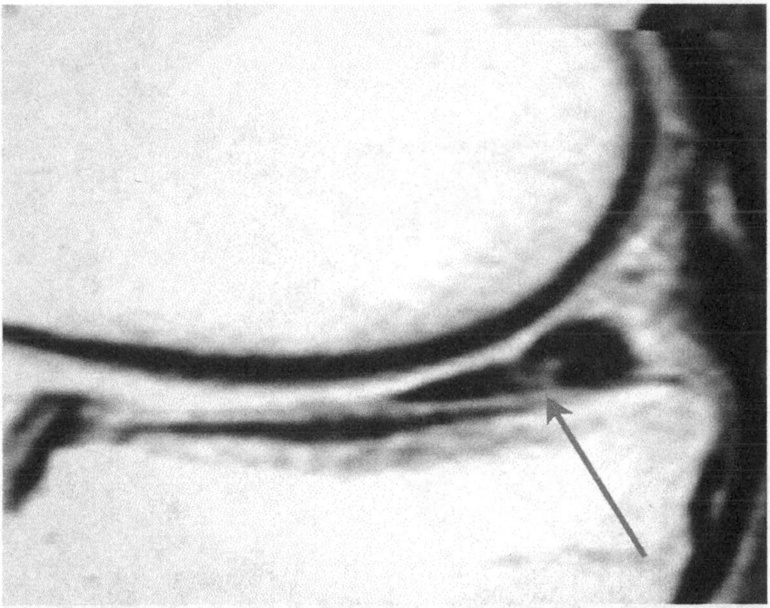

Figure 3-3. True meniscal tear on an MRI. The arrow points to the cleft between the meniscal fragments.

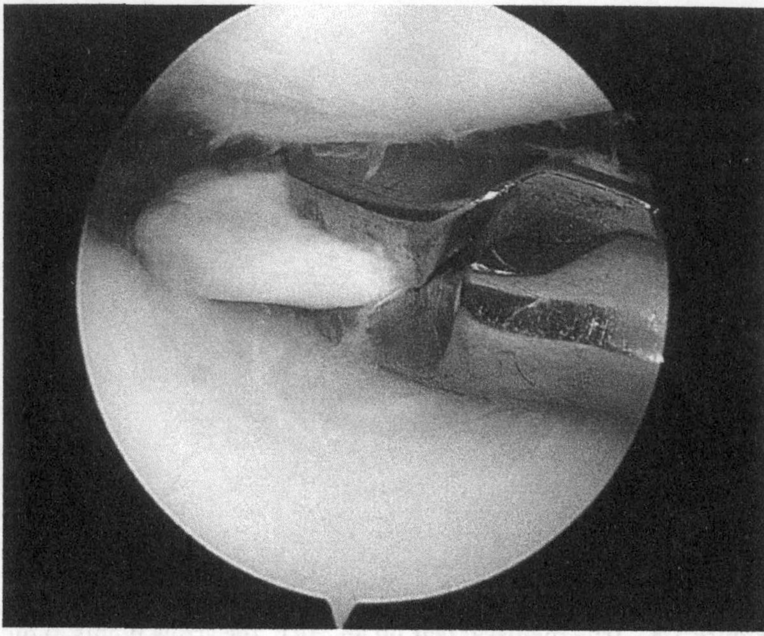

Figure 3-4. An arthroscopy "biter" is removing a flap tear.

CHAPTER 4
Stamp Out Torn Ligaments

Summary Soundbite:

- Not all ACL tears require surgery.

Case 1: Jane is skiing in soft snow when suddenly she catches the tip of her ski and feels a sharp pain in the left knee. The doctor says that she needs an MRI and ligament reconstruction—soon.

Case 2: Bill lands awkwardly from a jump and feels a painful pop in the right knee. The doctor informs him that he has a torn ACL and needs surgery—tomorrow.

Is this good advice?

A ligament is a sophisticated biological rope connecting two bones.[2] Some joints are quite solid ("stable"), and the ligaments are somewhat expendable. The hip joint, which consists of a large ball in a deep socket, is an example of such a joint. Even with a few ligaments removed, the hip ball does not readily come out of its socket. The knee and shoulder are at the other extreme. The knee can be likened to two large knobs resting on a flat surface; without ligaments, this structure would be completely unstable. The thigh bone would slide off the shinbone as would a ball off the end of a table. In a patient this would translate to the knee giving out.

[2] A tendon links a muscle to a bone.

There are four ligaments in and about the knee:

- The medial collateral ligament (MCL)
- The lateral (or fibular) collateral ligament (LCL)
- The posterior cruciate ligament (PCL)
- The anterior cruciate ligament (ACL) (the ligament the orthopedist most commonly gets to operate on)

The medial and lateral collateral ligaments lie relatively close to the skin on the inner and outer parts of the knee, respectively. The medial collateral ligament (MCL) is the most commonly injured ligament in the knee. It is injured when the upper leg is straight while the lower leg is rotated outward, as when catching the tip of a ski or when the knee is struck from the side as in a tackle (Figure 4-1). At the other extreme, the LCL resting on the outside of the knee is rarely injured.

Water on the knee. People with knee pain commonly feel that the knee is warm and swollen even if the heat is not detectable and the swelling is not visible to an outside observer. However, some patients truly have visible swelling, and this is particularly true in someone who has twisted his or her knee. When the knee is swollen, the orthopedist will want to differentiate between a knee that is simply puffy and a knee that is filled like a water balloon. A knee that is puffy is akin to a sponge that has absorbed water: if you put a needle in it, you will *not* get fluid out. This kind of swelling is common with any sprain, whether it be a knee, an ankle, or a finger injury. True water on the knee is a condition where fluid fills the joint in the same way that water fills a vase. The medical term for water on the knee is effusion. The knee *feels* like a water balloon. The "water" can simply be an excessive amount of so-called joint fluid, fluid that is present in every joint. Such fluid accumulation is not harmful.

People who suffer from arthritis are subject to this type of fluid collection. This is a reaction to the irritating byproducts of arthritis, and is the equivalent of an eye watering from a speck of dust. If one removes the fluid, it often comes right back. In the case of an injury though, the "water" can actually be blood. The presence of blood suggests to the doctor that the injury may in fact be more serious than a simple sprain. Removing excess blood from the joint can also alleviate some of the pain.

The medial collateral ligament (MCL)

The MCL can be injured with one of three degrees of severity (see Figure 4-2):

Grade I: The ligament is mildly stretched.

Grade II: The ligament has been considerably stretched but it is still in one piece.

Grade III: The ligament has been stretched and torn into two pieces. (Figure 4-2).

Each of these is very painful, and because of this, most people readily accept the concept that they have suffered a serious injury requiring an MRI and an operation. Wrong!

Testing. By and large, an MCL injury is easily diagnosed by a physical examination and it does not require an MRI. But it *does* require a physical examination, and I would not try to diagnose this on your own. Only in an athlete with a strict time schedule is it essential to get an MRI right after the injury: indeed there is always the chance that other injuries, such as a torn cartilage, may not be evident on the initial physical examination.

For the large majority of people, though, the most reasonable (cost-effective) course is to let the initial symptoms of the injury quiet down. The knee is rehabilitated, and, over the next two weeks, the doctor can establish whether there seems to be more than meets the eye. To the unscrupulous doctor the MRI can be very useful. (See below.)

Treatment

Surgery is not necessary. On occasion, a severe grade III tear of the MCL may require surgical reconstruction, but this is the exception rather than the rule. Sometimes the LK-SS[3] surgeon recommends an arthroscopic surgery just to make sure there is nothing else injured that might need fixing. Beware: This is where the unethical doctor will order an MRI and then recommend surgery based on the torn cartilage reported by the radiologist. As noted in the previous chapters, a so-called torn cartilage is a common finding in normal knees and does not automatically indicate the need for surgery. (The key word here is "automatically." Obviously, there are times when a person can have a true [grade III] tear requiring surgery.)

As with any injury, your doctor will recommend the application of cold packs the first forty-eight hours followed by the use of heat. The cold helps to minimize swelling, most of which will have occurred by forty-eight hours. Cold can be in the form of an ice pack or a gel pack that has been placed in the freezer. Cold packs should not be applied directly to the skin, as believe it or not, you can get frostbite! Rather, place a thin towel between the cold pack and the skin. Even better: obtain an elastic wrap (e.g., Ace®), wrap it once around the knee, place the ice pack against the elastic, and finish wrapping the elastic around the cold pack. This way you don't have to hold the cold pack in place. Best yet: a surgical supply store can probably sell you a Neoprene®-type sleeve equipped with pockets and gel packs. Once they are cold, just put the gel packs in the pockets and fasten the sleeve. In this setting (i.e., that of an injury) I would apply the cold pack around the clock—to the extent that it is practical for you. If the pack won't stay on while you are sleeping, don't deprive yourself of sleep just to apply an ice pack.

It is best not to use heat during the first forty-eight hours because contrary to cold, it may increase the swelling. Once the forty-eight hours are up, this is no longer an issue. It is soothing and it helps you bend and straighten that painful knee. You can use the same gel packs you'd been using for cold. Simply place them in hot water rather than in the freezer. Heating pads are acceptable, but don't fall asleep on them! Burns can occur. Dry

[3] LK-SS: Limited Knowledge–Suspect Scruples. See Chapter 1.

heat or moist heat? It doesn't matter. Use what works best for you. There is no limit to how long you should apply the heat.

Little secret: every now and then, even after the forty-eight hours are up, re-apply the cold pack. It's a good pain killer.

Going back and forth between heat and cold is not a problem.

Work on completely straightening the knee and bending it. You won't break anything. An injured knee wants to stay in a slightly bent position and doesn't want to be moved from that position. If you let it be, it will stiffen and tend to get stuck in that position. This stiffness may not be permanent, but it might take quite a bit of physical therapy to get rid of.

How much pain should you be in? The first twenty-four to forty-eight hours are painful, and you will want a narcotic such as codeine, oxycodone, or hydrocodone that the doctor can prescribe (unless you have addiction issues, in which case ask your doctor about tramadol). The narcotic masks the pain and there is nothing wrong with that in this setting! Narcotics can make you drowsy and/ or constipated. It's not a bad idea to take fruit juice, even milk of magnesia, or some other laxative. This approach works best before the problem sets in.

Note that besides relieving rest pain, pain medications allow you to perform the bending and straightening exercises described above.

In addition to narcotics, I recommend taking an anti-inflammatory medication unless there is a medical contraindication to this. This type of medication is abbreviated NSAID for "non-steroidal anti-inflammatory drug." You probably think that the anti-inflammatory medication will affect the swelling. It will not. The anti-inflammatory medication cuts down the pain and swelling at the microscopic level and diminishes pain by reducing the chemical irritation that takes place after an injury. Like Army and Navy, the narcotics and the anti-inflammatory medications complement each other. In this situation, they should be used in tandem. Anti-inflammatory medications are available over-the-counter in a weaker form. I would ask your doctor exactly how much you should take, or have him or her give you a prescription. There are medications that combine a narcotic and an anti-inflammatory drug, but as of this writing, these are brand rather than generic products and they tend to be considerably more expensive.

Relative medical contraindications to anti-inflammatory drugs include gastrointestinal ulcers, kidney dysfunction, bleeding disorders, the taking of blood thinners, and of course allergies (or intolerance) to specific anti-inflammatories.

As long as you are not suffering from side effects, you can take the NSAID medication for the few weeks that your knee can be expected to be painful. As the knee feels better you can gradually taper the frequency with which you take the medication.

- <u>Brand versus generic medications.</u> I am surprised by the number of doctors who prescribe new, brand name (i.e., expensive) anti-inflammatory medication as their first choice. Clearly they aren't paying for them! By and large, there is no difference in efficacy between a new NSAID and one whose patent has run out. Time-tested anti-inflammatory medications include naproxen, ibuprofen, and diclofenac—to name a few. The patents have long run out on these medications, and they are no longer promoted in their original form by their parent company. They are certainly effective, and you are not likely to wake up tomorrow to find that they have been pulled off the market. For the majority of people with knee pain, one of these medications should be prescribed first.

  NSAIDs can be differentiated from each other mainly by their strength and by their half-life (a measure of how long the drug stays in your body). For example, ibuprofen is short acting and needs to be taken three or four times a day to be effective around the clock. Piroxicam is at the other extreme: it just needs to be taken once day. On the other hand, ibuprofen works faster and is therefore preferable when someone is injured and requires quick relief. The prescription dose of ibuprofen is 600 mg three to four times a day (less in older people).

- Cox-2 inhibitors. These block one of the chemicals that cause pain without blocking the chemicals that protect the stomach.

  Thus, in theory, they are less likely to cause stomach ulcers and bleeding than the more traditional anti-inflammatory medications. Until their patent runs out, these NSAIDs will be rather expensive and, in my opinion, should be reserved for people who are at risk for ulcers. This includes people over fifty-five to sixty years of age and those with a history of stomach problems. Know that controversy exists as to just how effective these Cox-2 inhibitors are at protecting the stomach.

  Issues have been raised with respect to the cardiac safety of certain NSAIDs taken over long periods of time, and I would discuss this with your doctor if you're going to be on long-term anti-inflammatories.
- Acetaminophen (Tylenol®). Once the pain of the injury has quieted down, this can be a very effective (and cost-effective) medication. It can be taken with an NSAID. In fact, when an NSAID is allowed, I recommend adding acetaminophen. It attacks pain by way of a different chemical path and complements that of an NSAID (see my Army-Navy analogy in the narcotic section above). Many narcotic preparations include acetaminophen (e.g., Tylenol #3®, Vicodin®, Percocet®, Norco®), a testament to its efficacy.

  On the negative side, narcotic preparations that contain quite a bit of acetaminophen can lead to acetaminophen toxicity. If you are taking one of those (e.g., Vicodin®), discuss this issue with your doctor.
- Ultram® (Tramadol). This pain reliever is in a category by itself. It is neither an NSAID nor a narcotic, and it is stronger than acetaminophen. A small percentage of patients develop dizziness and should stop it; for patients who tolerate it though, it is a good choice.
- Braces. Although no bone is broken when an MCL is torn, it can sure feel that way. A brace can make it less painful to put the foot on the ground. You need a brace with firm plastic or

metallic stays along the sides that can be found in a surgical supply store (a store that sells canes, crutches, and the like). The brace should cost around a hundred dollars but may or may not be reimbursed by your insurance plan.

Phase 1 (first week or two). Initially, the best brace to apply is a so-called "knee immobilizer" which goes from the top of the thigh down to the ankle. As the name implies, it does not allow the knee to bend. It fastens with Velcro® straps and is therefore easy to put on and remove. You will need it most when you walk, and you will probably also want to use it at night, as simply catching your foot on the sheets can be quite painful. It can be removed when you sit, when you want to bend the knee, or when you wash.

Beware: immobilizers come in different lengths, from approximately twelve to twenty-four inches. If your immobilizer is too long it will dig into your groin and/or irritate your ankle. If it is too short, it won't adequately support you and will not provide adequate pain relief. Ideally, the immobilizer should start at the upper thigh and come down to two inches above your anklebone. Some immobilizers have built-in pouches for hot and cold gel packs, and this is beneficial.

Certain immobilizers feature a locking-unlocking hinge. (Technically, they are no longer called immobilizers but braces.) The patient can lock the hinge when he or she wishes support (as when walking), and can unlock it when looking to bend the knee (as when sitting). Such braces will cost $200 to $300 and again, will only be necessary for ten days to two weeks. Is the extra convenience worth the cost? Not for most people—at least not those paying out of pocket.

Phase 2. As the pain subsides over the two weeks following the injury, you will no longer need the knee immobilizer, but you will still benefit from some support. A hinged brace is now ideal: this is a somewhat short brace, which features a hinge on both sides of the knee. The hinge allows the knee to bend while protecting the knee from side-to-side forces. Such forces can be expected to remain painful for at least another month or two.

The return to sports

This is simple: you can return when you are up to it. The knee should be pain-free and should come close to having regained its normal strength and coordination. Naturally, the more severe the injury, the longer it will take. The mildest sprains keep you out about three weeks, the more severe ones about three to six months. At first you will wear the hinged brace during sports, and gradually you will wean yourself from it. Sports involving little or no twisting will be easier to resume. Running, biking, jumping rope, and swimming are easier (and safer) to engage in than football, basketball, squash, volleyball, or tennis. For tennis players, clay-type surfaces are more friendly than concrete since the foot is less likely to stick to the ground when the body and leg turn.

Prevention

A ligament is a very special rope, but nevertheless it is a rope. Therefore it is difficult to condition it. On the other hand, the knee is also surrounded by strong muscles. With proper conditioning these muscles can be strengthened and programmed to react quickly. Therefore, the muscles help control the knee and can diminish the chance of an MCL tear.

The use of a hinged brace (see above) should also decrease the chance of an MCL injury and is recommended for people who have already injured this ligament. Athletes most at risk are skiers and football players. Generally, though, the use of knee braces to prevent injury is controversial. I formally recommend this only to athletes who are ginger from a prior injury.

Skiers tend to injure their knees on the proverbial last run of the day. This saying has always amused me because any kind of knee injury turns a ski run into a "last run." It is true, however, that the majority of ski injuries occur late in the day. When we ran a sports clinic at the base of Hunter Mountain in New York, the late afternoon was always the busiest time. There are numerous reasons for this including a flatter light, icier conditions, and greater fatigue. Muscles tire and become less able to quickly contract and protect ligaments such as the MCL. Therefore, "quit while you're ahead" remains a good adage for injury prevention.

A conditioning program is useful for both treatment and prevention. This starts with stretching (See Figure 4-3 and Figures in Chapter 11).

When observed under a microscope, ligaments and tendons look like spring-like coils. Through slow and steady tension, these springs can be partially uncoiled. The operative phrase here is "slow and steady." Tension which is strong and sudden will simply result in tearing the structure, which is what happens in an injury. A stretch should be held twenty seconds to effectively elongate those little coils.

The more these so-called soft tissues are stretched prior to athletics, the less likely they are likely to snap when they are suddenly stressed. The structures in the front of the knee are stretched by bringing the heel to the buttock with the hip in the extended (non-bent) position, and this exercise can be carried out in the standing position (See Figure 4-3). The structures in the back of the thigh (hamstrings) are stretched by touching the toes without bending the knees. This can be done standing or sitting on the ground. Careful: this maneuver also stretches another important rope—the sciatic nerve. This nerve runs from the spine, down the buttock, and down the back of the leg. A healthy nerve can be gently stretched in the manner described, but a sciatic nerve that is irritated for any reason will not take kindly to this type of expansion. Therefore stretching of the hamstrings should not be carried out if pain ensues.

More sophisticated stretching involves the IT band (iliotibial band) that runs along the outside of the leg. The inside part of the leg is addressed by way of stretching the adductors, the muscles that run along the inside of the thigh. The adductors are also subject to sudden stretching injuries when a person lunges to the side, as when reaching for a tennis ball. The adductors, therefore, deserve to be part of any stretching program (see Chapter 11).

The Anterior Cruciate Ligament (ACL)

This remains a very fashionable ligament. Mention an ACL injury at a cocktail party, and you receive grave nods of approval. Everybody recognizes this as an athlete's injury, and an ACL tear puts you in the category of the elite skiers, football players, and basketball players. You might even have one of those large, glitzy knee braces that come in any number of designer patterns and colors. If you're a teenager, you'll demand one.

The historical perspective. The pendulum often swings one way and then the other before a happy medium is reached. Until thirty-forty years ago, the medical profession did not take ACL injuries very seriously. There were four reasons for this:

1. Neither MRIs nor arthroscopies were common, leading a number of tears to be altogether missed.
2. ACL-deficient athletes either felt perfectly well or at most had a trick knee—a knee that "goes in and out" when the leg is turned in a certain way. In short, most people could (and still can) live with a torn ACL, and indeed have done so since the beginning of time.
3. There were no apparent long-term problems associated with this injury.
4. There were no effective operations.

We now know that in an athlete a torn ACL predisposes the knee to further meniscal (cartilage) tears and can lead to arthritis. Moreover, the ACL can currently be reconstructed without resorting to lengthy incisions about the knee. This has all led to a remarkable flurry of ACL surgery, some of which is unnecessary (see below).

Where is the ACL and what does it do?

As noted at the beginning of this chapter, the knee is inherently unstable: it is totally dependent on ligaments and other soft tissues to stay in place. Contrary to the MCL which runs close to the skin, the ACL lies deep inside the knee. It courses obliquely from the outer part of the thighbone at the back of the knee down to the table-like portion of the upper shinbone, the tibial plateau) (Figures 4-4a, b, and c). The ACL prevents the knee from hyperextending (bending backward) and from becoming unhinged during certain twisting motions.

The ACL can be likened to a cable made of many strands. These strands are visible to the naked eye and can be seen to subtly twist around each other. There is some elasticity to these fibers and therefore some give when the knee is pushed too far. Some people are loose-jointed, and by definition, their ligaments tend to have more stretch. They are less likely to tear their ACL, but conversely, in the event of such an injury, the other ligaments are less able to pick up the slack.

How do you injure an ACL?

By and large it requires a significant injury to tear an ACL. You don't tear an ACL while getting up from the floor as you might a meniscus (see Chapter 3). The foot has to be planted, and the knee has to be twisted during hyperextension or hyperflexion (over-straightening or bending). Skiing, soccer, and football produce these injuries. The typical ski injury involves falling or sitting onto the back of a ski as the tip of the ski veers off to the side. Tackling in football, soccer, rugby and related sports can lead to a tear of the ACL. Generally speaking, it takes more force to tear an ACL than an MCL, but on occasion, ACL tears have been seen to occur *without* significant trauma in athletes who suddenly pivot as they run (the so-called atraumatic ACL tear). The athlete with a torn ACL usually feels a pop and/or notices rapid and painful swelling; weight-bearing on the affected is difficult; crutches are usually required. If fluid is drained from the knee, it is usually bloody.

On examination, the tibia (shinbone) can be pulled forward. This is called the drawer maneuver or the Lachman depending on whether the knee is bent or straight when the test is carried out.

The doctor may also try a pivot test whereby the tibia snaps in and out of place as the knee is gently flexed and twisted back and forth.

Can you prevent an ACL injury?

By training for a particular activity you can decrease the odds of suffering an ACL injury, but you cannot eliminate the risk. High-level athletes tear this ligament with alarming frequency. No brace protects a knee from this injury, and if it existed, it would probably be too cumbersome and expensive to be prescribed on a routine basis.

However, there now exist ACL prevention programs. (See below.) In the skiing world, sitting back on one's skis is a known risk factor—and of course this is a natural reaction on the part of any beginner skier.

Why are women more at risk?

One hears surprisingly little about this on a daily basis, even though there have been numerous scientific articles and presentations about this subject. The issue of women's increased risk for major ligament injuries has even been a featured article in *Sports Illustrated* magazine.

Women have been found to be at particular risk in basketball and soccer. Other sports have been less thoroughly evaluated. Depending on the study and the setting in which women were being followed, women have been found to be anywhere from three to ten times more at risk for a tear of the ACL than men.

Theories for the discrepancy between men and women have centered on joint laxity, hormonal variations with the menstrual cycle, reaction times (how quickly muscles react to an event), and body position during jumping and landing. Strength per se does not seem to be an issue. In my experience, women and girls who participate in these sports are not fully aware of their particular risk for an ACL tear, that is, they and their parents are not informed consumers. This a particular concern in younger women since they are the ones most likely to need surgery. In some circles, it is politically incorrect to even bring up the subject.

ACL prevention programs geared toward girls and women have now been developed; their focus tends to be on body position when landing from a jump, as women tend to be more stiff-kneed upon landing. I recommend an Internet search of "ACL prevention programs" along with the search terms "American Society of Orthopedic Surgeons" (or AAOS) and "American Orthopaedic Society for Sports Medicine" (or AOSSM).

Do you need surgery?

A number of you will have zoomed right to this section. If you've had an ACL injury this is what is uppermost in your mind. And the answer is . . . it depends. If you are an adolescent the answer is unequivocally yes, though you might wait until you've just about stopped growing. (See below.) The answer is also "yes" if you perform jumping/twisting activities, since the ACL is a major stabilizer of the knee in those situations. The same holds if your knee is *unstable* as a result of the injury. (Patients will commonly move one fist over the other to demonstrate that feeling.) This used to be called a trick knee.

At the other extreme, if you are over forty years old, symptom-free, and all your athletic activities are of the low impact, straight-ahead variety such as cycling, swimming, and intermediate hiking, surgery is not necessary. Everyone in-between presents a dilemma. You have to weigh the risk of surgery against the risk of perhaps damaging more structures in your knee (which then increases your risk of arthritis).

Indeed, the abnormal mechanics of the knee which result from the injury can, in some people, lead to arthritis (wearing out of the articular cartilage). As of this writing, the medical profession is not able to predict who will and who will not develop arthritis as a result of an ACL tear. The following seem to be risk factors: associated tears of a meniscus (also known as cartilage; see Chapter 3). If a large piece of the meniscus has to be removed, the knee is that much less stable. When this instability is added to that caused by the ACL tear, the combination appears to be too much for the knee to handle, and arthritis ensues two or more decades down the road.

Another risk factor appears to be a bone bruise seen on an MRI. Such a bruise indicates that the knee took a significant hit at the time of the injury. A bruise can lead to a "hot" bone scan. (The test is formally called a nuclear three-phase technetium scan.) For this test, a lightly radioactive material is injected intravenously. The technetium is mainly absorbed by bony tissue. When much of it is absorbed in one (hot) spot, it indicates greater than normal bony activity. In the setting of an ACL tear, the hot spot reflects the body's attempt to repair the bony damage that was incurred at the time of the ACL tear. Some orthopedists feel that these bruises in and of themselves lead to an increased risk of arthritis. If this is correct, reconstructing the ACL of patients with bone bruises may not prevent arthritis![4] Welcome to the convoluted world of ACL tears.

On occasion, the ligament is partially torn: it appears slightly stretched or only some of the fibers appear torn. When the tear only involves a few wisps of ligament, no reconstruction is required. But with larger tears there can be a treatment dilemma: leave it or reconstruct it? The surgeon has to determine whether the reconstructed ligament will be better than your imperfect ACL. I tend to err on leaving the patient's own ligament unless the patient's symptoms can only be explained by the partial tear.

If you fall into this large group of borderline patients, only you can make the decision of whether to have surgery or not. There is no right answer, only what is right for you. Whichever road you choose, you should embark upon it with confidence. You will be happier with the results.

---

[4] A number of studies have suggested that ACL reconstruction does not prevent arthritis in anyone.

When should surgery be performed?

Is it better to operate on the knee when it has just been seriously traumatized or is it better to wait for the knee to have recovered somewhat before assaulting it again? You can argue this all day. Needless to say, orthopedists in ski resorts see things somewhat differently from their colleagues in the cities. As a city orthopedist, I would rather let the athlete adjust to the physical and emotional aspect of the trauma, let him or her collect their wits, search the Internet, make the appropriate work/school arrangements, rehab the knee to get reasonable strength and motion back, and then peacefully and carefully reconstruct the ligament. In cities, as in mountains resorts, a number of orthopedists use the shoe salesman approach described in the previous chapter: sign up the patient for surgery right away, or risk losing the patient. After all, a few weeks later the patient may feel well and refuse surgery altogether.

ACL injuries in adolescents

This is not as controversial as it used to be. Children who have an ACL that has been torn have a bleak knee future. The difficulty lies in the choice of surgery: all accepted procedures in adults involve making holes in bones about the knee, and this happens to be where the major growth plates are in adolescents. Surgery performed through growth plates has the potential to affect bony growth. This is particularly critical in children with much growth left, and is of lesser importance to those whose growth is nearly complete. Ideally then, the surgeon should wait until the child has nearly stopped growing, and there are ways for the doctor to assess a child's anticipated growth. However, this means holding the child back from certain sports—usually a nonstarter.

Current surgical options *all* avoid the placement of screws within a growth plate, but the orthopedic community has yet to agree on one specific operation or type of fixation.

Types of surgery

When something is torn and the ends have pulled apart, the natural reaction is to sew them back together. Not surprisingly then, the earliest operations for a torn ACL consisted of sewing the ACL back together. This did not work. Perhaps the techniques were inadequate or perhaps a stretched and torn cablelike structure is simply not amenable to sewing. In any case, the current party line is that by and large, a completely (or even mostly) torn ACL cannot be fixed.

Thermal shrinkage does not work either. It was promoted over ten years ago as a way to tighten fibers that are stretched but not torn. The surgeon simply touches the ACL with a hot wand and the fibers crinkle up. It seemed like a good idea at the time; certainly, it was easy. Alas, it appears that the fibers uncrinkle. For some surgeons, unfortunately, this approach continues to be irresistible. (See "How to Interpret Your Arthroscopy Report" at the end of Chapter 3.)

If the ACL is deficient, it needs to be reconstructed with another structure. This structure can be from your own body (an autograft), it can come from a bone bank—an elegant way of saying that it comes from a cadaver (an allograft), or it can be synthetic. Synthetics are naturally the most appealing, but those that have been tried in the United States have not worked.

Types of graft:

- Patellar tendon ("bone-patellar-bone")
- Gracilis / Semi-tendinosis ("hamstring")
- Quadriceps tendon
- Allograft

Allografts have the obvious advantage over autografts of leaving your own body intact; you're not sacrificing any part of your body. But cadaveric allografts are expensive, they are not always available, and more significantly, there is always the small chance that some disease will be transmitted. With your luck the cadaver will have had some hidden, horrible disease, right? Because of this small chance, grafts are heavily radiated to the point where cynics have likened them to a piece of bacon. That's not really fair, but the point is that allografts are an acceptable but not ideal solution.

Indications for an allograft: Allografts tend to be used when multiple grafts are needed, when a quicker recovery is desired, when the patient is going for a reoperation (and an autograft has already been used), or simply when neither the patient nor the surgeon wants to "rob Peter to pay Paul." (All autografts by definition sacrifice healthy tendons.)

In the future we can expect to either grow a new ligament or find an acceptable synthetic ligament. In the meantime, there are three main sources of autografts: the patellar tendon, the hamstring tendons, and the quadriceps tendon.

The patellar tendon graft consists of the middle third of the tendon connecting your kneecap (patella) to your tibial tuberosity (the knob at the top of your shinbone), as well as a piece of bone at each end of the tendon. One piece of bone comes off the kneecap and the other comes off the tuberosity (see Figure 4-2b). You would think that this would leave the rest of the patellar tendon quite weakened and prone to rupture, but with cautious rehabilitation that has not been the case. This is fortunate because a rupture of the patellar tendon is close to an orthopedic disaster requiring at the very least one major operation and a long period of recovery.

Once the graft is harvested, it has to be placed inside the knee. For this, holes ("tunnels") are created, and the graft is passed into those holes. The graft has to be locked into the first tunnel, made taut, and finally, fixed to the other tunnel (Figure 4-3). The advantage of having a piece of bone at either end of the graft is that a screw can be placed in the tunnels, thus wedging the bone from the graft to the walls of the tendon. Bone heals well to bone. So-called soft tissue screws are also available. These permit screw fixation of soft tissues, such as hamstring or quadriceps tendon grafts. Within a few months, the graft is forever secured.

Unfortunately, as Hall of Famer Jerry Rice of the San Francisco 49ers will attest to (he broke his kneecap one day after returning to football), the fact that the graft has healed does not mean that the recovery is over. The host site—the place that the graft was taken from—needs time to recover. In the case of a patellar tendon graft, if stressed too soon or too vigorously, the kneecap may fracture, or the remaining tendon may rupture. The rope that was just placed in the knee also needs time to start looking and acting like an ACL. Opinions are divided with regards to how long this takes. Some say two years, but nobody wants to wait that long. The party line is one year. One year therefore before resuming contact sports.

The very long-term effects of harvesting an autograft of any kind are not known.

<u>The hamstring graft.</u> You have three hamstring muscles running down the back of your thigh: the biceps (yes, same as in your arm); the semitendinosus and the semimembranosus. In the hamstring graft, the semitendinosus is harvested, often along with the gracilis tendon running along the inner thigh (See Figure 4-6). These tendons are there for a purpose, so for the surgeon it is emotionally painful to sacrifice them. Yet, athletes appear to function well even after these tendons are harvested. There is less donor site morbidity, as we say in medical lingo, than with harvesting of the patellar tendon: nothing bad is going to happen to the site from which the graft was taken if the athlete makes a hasty return to sports.

As with all grafts, there are umpteen ways of fixing a hamstring graft to the bone, but they all involve so-called hardware—a screw, a staple, and so forth. Some of this hardware can be absorbable; instead of being metallic, it is made of a dissolvable material. These products are still evolving (See Figure 4-6b).

The quadriceps tendon graft. The quadriceps tendon joins the quadriceps muscles at the front of your thigh to the kneecap. It has some of the advantages and disadvantages of the other two grafts and is equally acceptable. In the United States, this graft is uncommon.

At the present, a surgeon's comfort level with a certain graft is probably more important than the graft itself.

Rehabilitation

In the old days (up until forty years ago), people undergoing ligament surgery were placed in a long-leg cast. Not only was it terribly inconvenient, but it was unnecessary and harmful. Today, therapy starts right away. Normal bending and straightening is of the utmost importance. This is not so easy because the operated knee generally does not want to move; it likes to stay slightly bent and left alone. What else happens when the knee hurts? Muscles tend to atrophy and tendons tighten up. The therapist works with you to reverse that process.

The best way to train for a certain activity is to perform exercises that simulate that activity. Therefore, isokinetic exercises whereby you sit in a chair and straighten your leg against a resistance are of limited value after the initial recovery phase. The same holds for the use of an exercise bicycle. Regardless of where you get your therapy (and yes, some form of physical therapy is essential), you should be progressing from motion exercises, to simple strengthening movements, to more sophisticated exercise routines. Eventually, the therapist elaborates a program for you that you can carry out at home or at the gym.

Return to sports

Some patients are satisfied with simply having a stable knee during everyday activities, but most patients with ACL tears want to go back to sports. Activities that put the reconstructed ligament at risk are the same ones that led to the ACL tear in the first place: uncontrolled jumping and twisting. These are therefore the last to be permitted. On the other hand, running, jumping in place with both feet, and even side-to-side jumping are allowed early on. Swimming is also admissible once the skin is healed.

Can the new, surgically reconstructed ACL rupture too?

You bet. A paradox of sports medicine is that we operate on knees so that athletes can go back to the sports they love, yet those very activities can lead to a rupture of the new ACL. Since the new ACL is a relatively crude version of the original, it is easier to tear than the original. And as with all operations, the surgery the second time around is far more complex than the first one. As bitter a pill as it is to swallow, the person who doesn't earn a living from sports might consider toning down his or her activities after an ACL reconstruction.

The Posterior Cruciate and Lateral (Fibular) Collateral Ligament

Injuries to these ligaments are far less common, but potentially far more serious. The posterior cruciate ligament (PCL) lies in the center of the knee where it crosses behind its anterior counterpart, the ACL. It shares some functions with the ACL to the extent that it helps provide smooth, controlled motion of the knee. It does so, however, in a manner just opposite the ACL, which is understandable considering that one goes from top right to bottom left, so to speak, and the other goes from top left to bottom right. The PCL prevents the thighbone from sliding forward when one goes down steps, and as with the ACL, it resists abnormal twisting.

The lateral collateral ligament (LCL), also called fibular collateral ligament, is the equivalent of the MCL: it lies relatively close to the skin along the outer aspect of the knee. In a manner similar to the MCL, it takes its origin on the femur, but instead of inserting on the upper tibia as does the MCL, it inserts at the top of the fibula, the skinny bone on the outer aspect of the leg.

Whereas the MCL is the most commonly injured ligament, the LCL is arguably the least commonly injured ligament. This is fortunate because when the LCL is torn, the PCL is commonly torn too (and vice versa), and this combination commonly mandates surgery: it will not heal on its own, and left untreated it will lead to a very unstable knee.

Isolated PCL tears are quite rare and the necessity to address this problem surgically is more controversial. Many patients with an isolated PCL tear do not even realize that they have a torn ligament. An isolated PCL tear can occur when the tibia is forcibly pushed backward. Landing with your shin on a log, for example, will push the shinbone backward relative to the knee. Rarely, hitting the knee against a dashboard will push the leg back in such a way as to tear the PCL (not the ACL). (This is not an excuse for getting an MRI on everyone who hits his/her knee on a dashboard.) An isolated PCL tear may be asymptomatic and therefore does not automatically mandate surgery. But in young, athletic people, a torn PCL probably leads to subtle abnormal motions and is probably best reconstructed. This was the injury sustained by the notable quarterback Randall Cunningham before his resounding comeback with the Minnesota Vikings. Note that once again, a PCL cannot be repaired, that is, stitched back together. As with the ACL, it needs to be reconstructed with another structure. Because the PCL tends to be torn along with other structures (ACL and/or LCL), chances are that an allograft will be used for part of the reconstruction. (See above paragraph on ACL surgery.)

Isolated LCL injuries are distinctly unusual and most of the time require surgery.

Fortunately, we live in an era where these injuries can be detected and a surgical solution, albeit imperfect, can be offered.

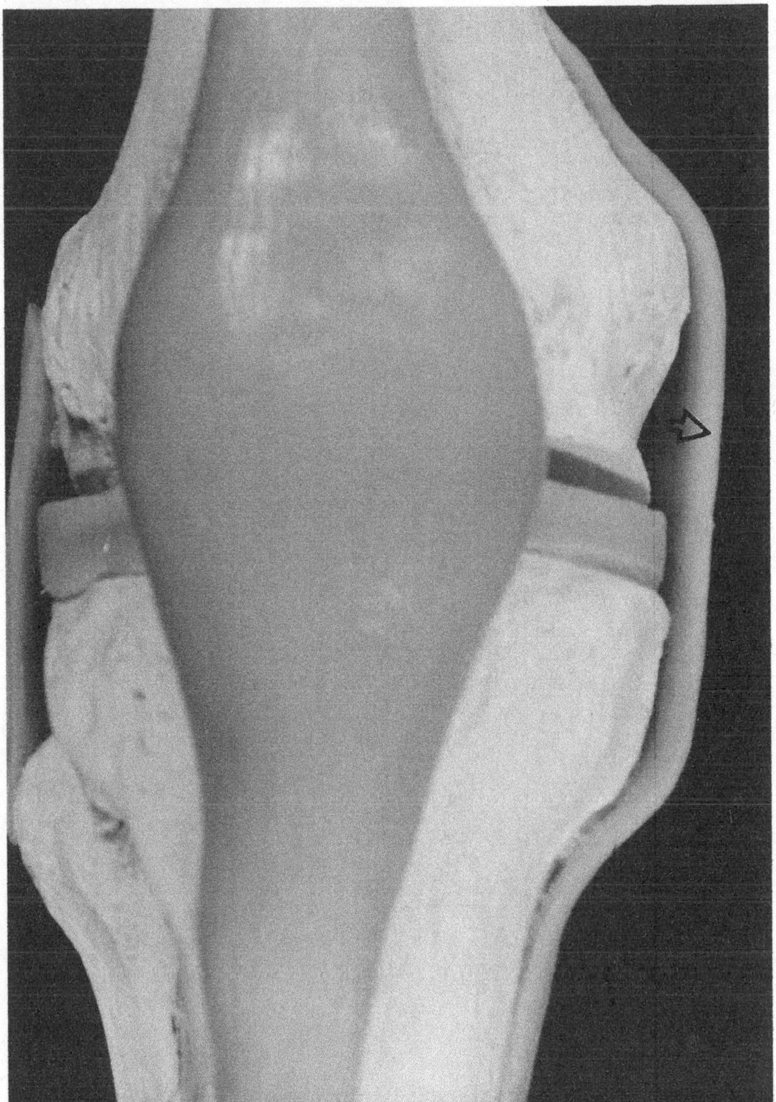

Figure 4-1. The medial collateral ligament (MCL). This ligament is commonly injured.

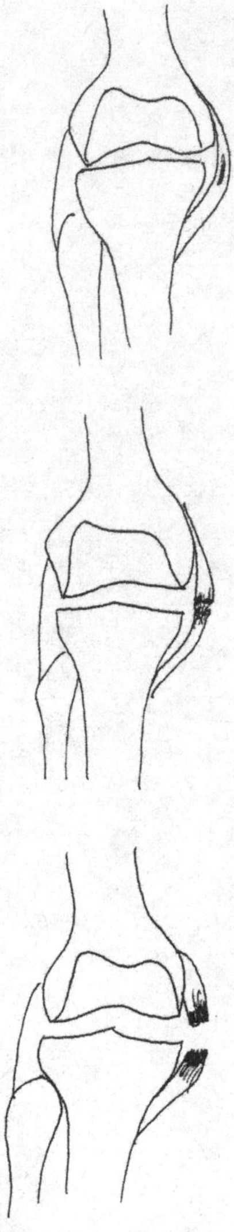

Figure 4-2. MCL injuries. Grade 1 (top); painful, but the knee is not rendered unstable. Grade 2 (middle); with each step the subject may feel some "give" in the knee. Grade 3 (bottom); unstable—with each step, the knee opens like a hinge.

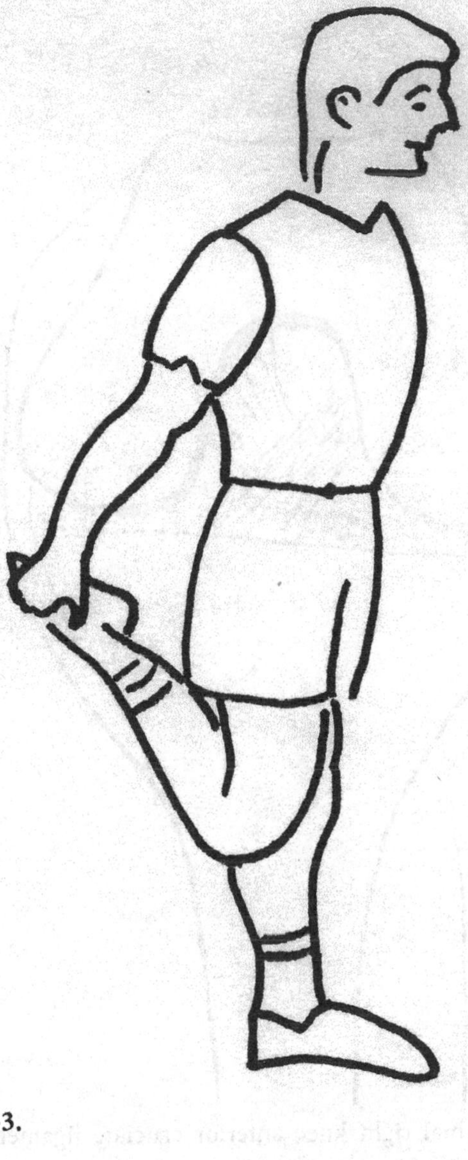

Figure 4-3.

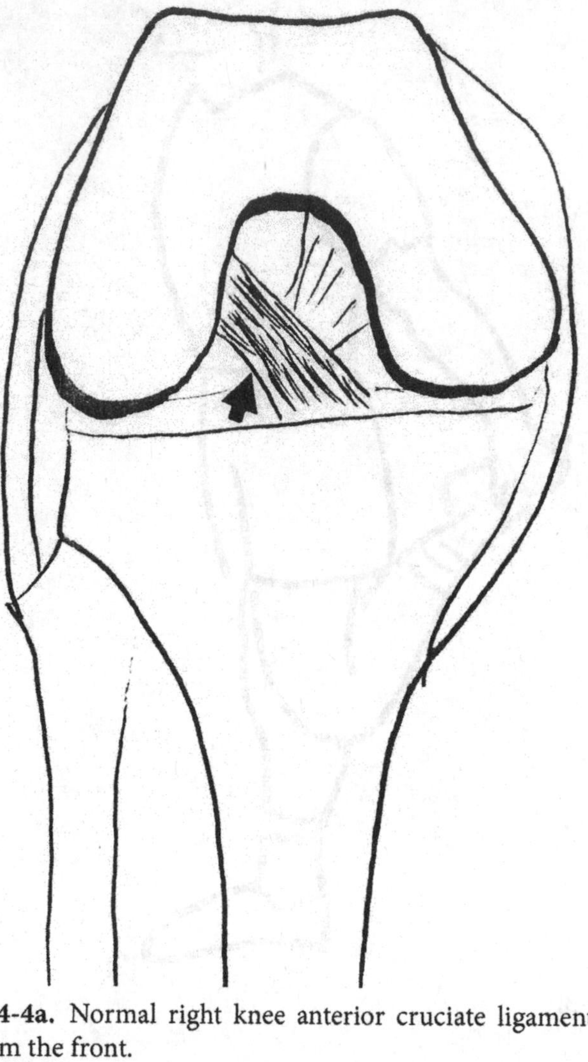

Figure 4-4a. Normal right knee anterior cruciate ligament (ACL) seen from the front.

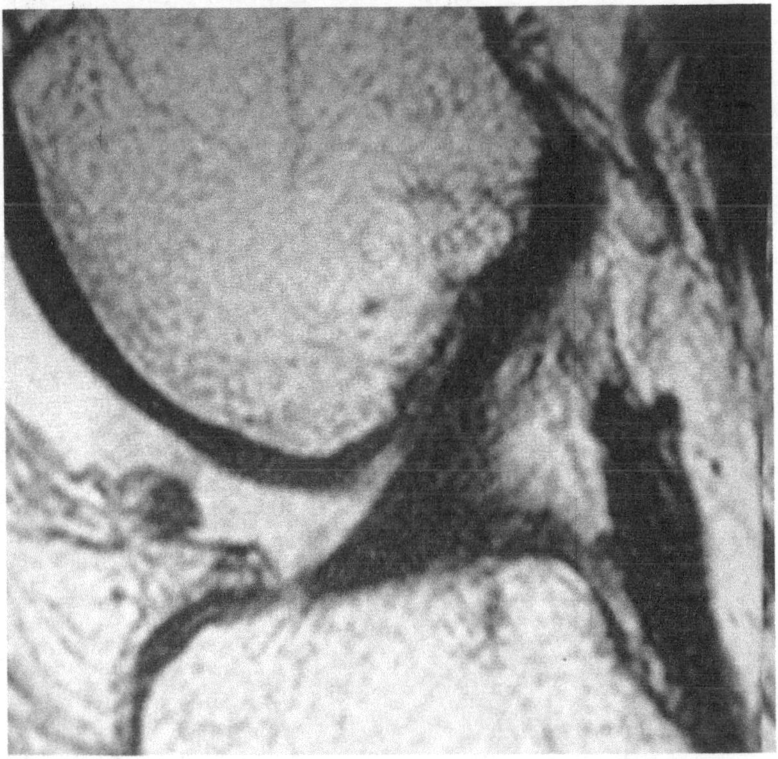

Figure 4-4b. A normal ACL as seen on a side-view of a knee MRI.

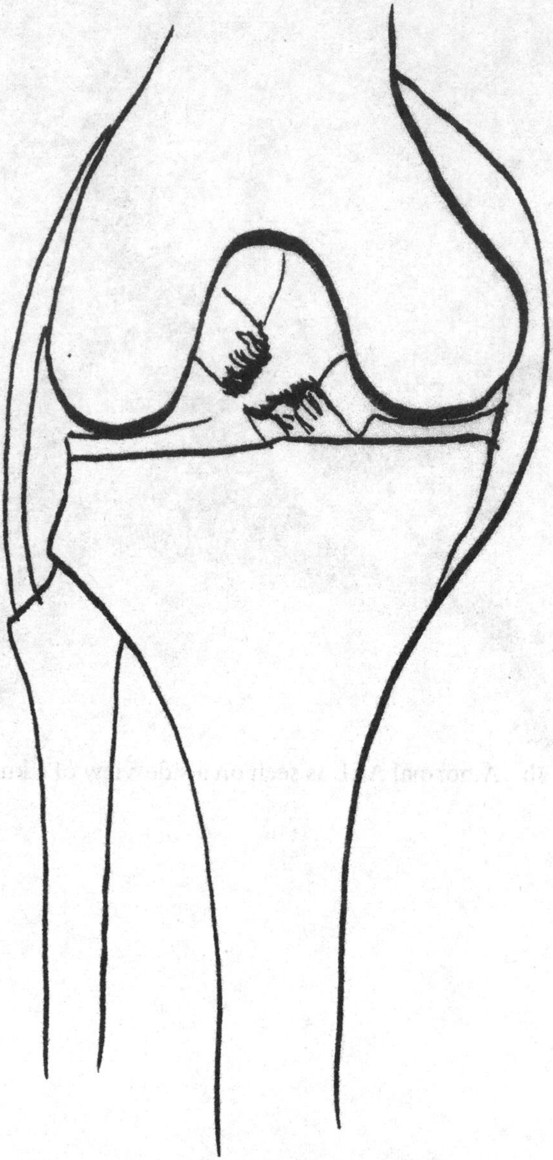

Figure 4-4c. A torn right ACL seen from the front.

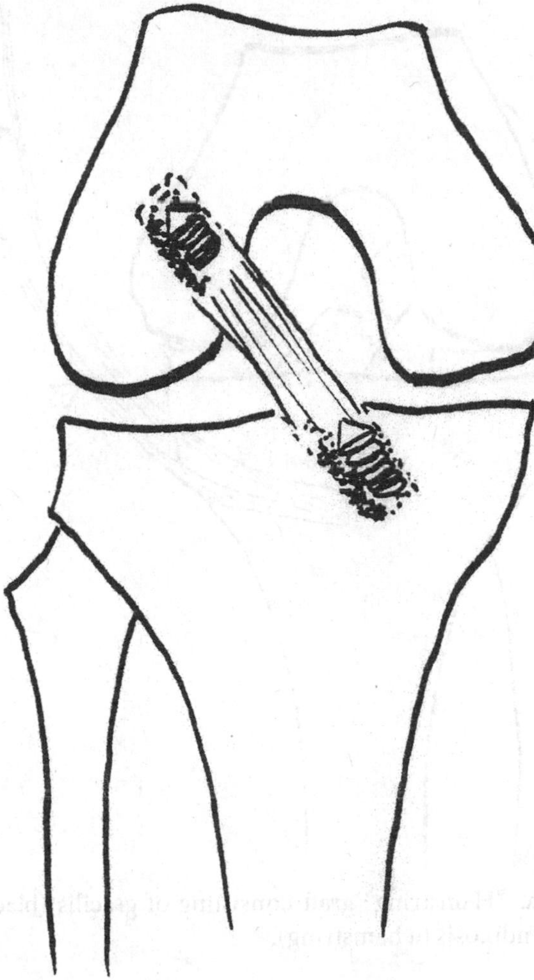

Figure 4-5c. Traditionally reconstructed right knee ACL viewed from the front. A screw fixes the graft in both the femur and the tibia. There are many variations on this.

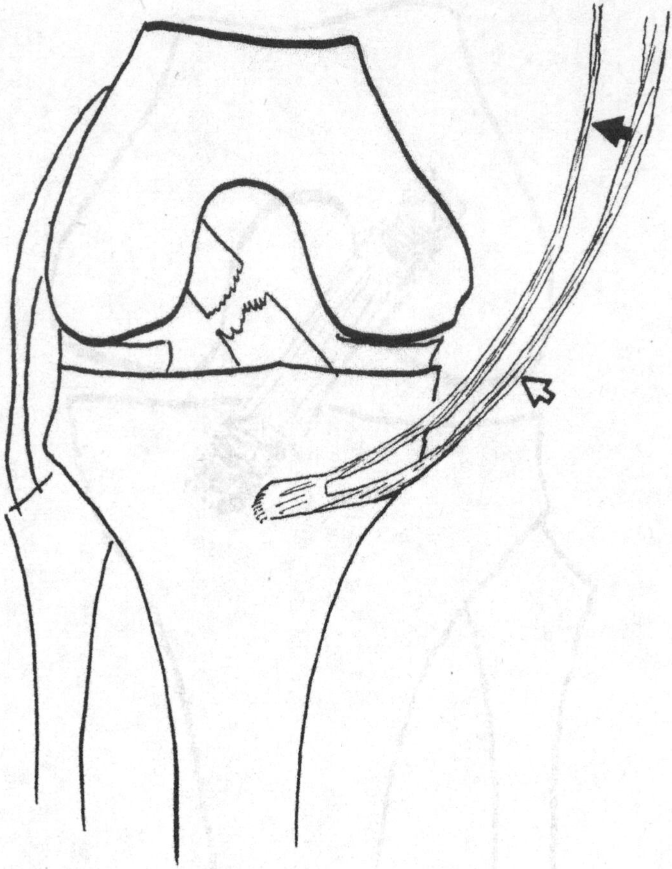

Figure 4-6a. "Hamstring" graft consisting of gracilis (black arrow) and semi-tendinosis (a hamstring).

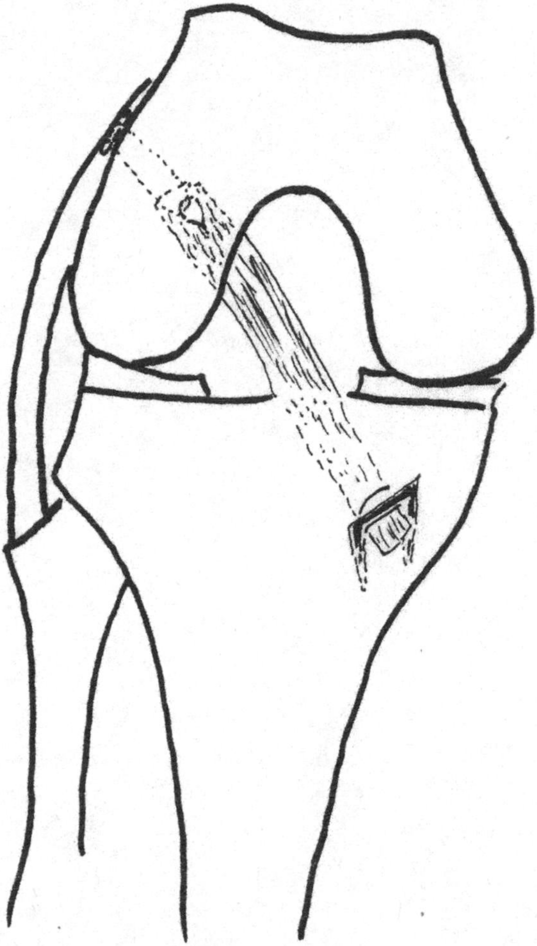

Figure 4-6b. Fixation of a "hamstring" graft. In this example, the femoral (upper) tunnel is fixed with a small metallic button and sophisticated rope while the (lower) tibial tunnel is fixed with a staple. As of this writing, the tibial portion is likely to be fixed with a screw. New methods of fixation are continuously introduced.

CHAPTER 5

"Urgent" Arthritis Surgery

Summary Soundbites:

- There are many treatment options prior to surgery.
- Little cleanup surgeries don't usually work—even in the presence of a torn meniscus

There is no urgent arthritis surgery. But that's not always the sense I get from patients. They've seen an orthopedist who's told them that the x-rays look bad and that they need surgery—soon.

What is arthritis?

A white, shiny material lines the end of each bone. Check it out the next time you eat chicken. This material is called cartilage. Specifically, it is articular cartilage. The term articular differentiates it from meniscal cartilage, the rubbery shock absorber described in Chapter 3. The term "torn cartilage" refers to meniscal cartilage.

Arthritis represents the wearing down of articular cartilage down to the bone (see Figure 5-1a and b).

Arthritis can have multiple causes. These include a genetically caused deterioration of the cartilage; a mechanical overload of the cartilage; as when people are very bow-legged, knock-kneed, and/or overweight; trauma—a fracture through the cartilage for example; an infection; or a rheumatological condition whereby the lining of the joint secretes a product that slowly degrades articular cartilage (see also Chapter 6).

Arthritis can involve just one small part of the knee or it can be more generalized.

The role of x-rays

There are four major misconceptions with regard to x-rays and arthritis:

Misconception #1. You really need an MRI, not an x-ray. Not true. In many cases, an x-ray is sufficient to make a diagnosis of arthritis (See Figure 5-2). It is upsetting to find patients coming into the office holding an MRI when an x-ray costing one-tenth the price would have sufficed. We are all paying for these tests!

Although cartilage does not show up on an x-ray, arthritis can be apparent in different ways. For example, the space between the bones becomes narrower (joint space narrowing), a sign that the cartilage is wearing thin. In extreme cases, the bones are seen to touch each other. This indicates that the cartilage is completely worn out. Another radiographic sign of arthritis is the presence of bone spurs called osteophytes. They tell the doctor, "Look over here, there's worn cartilage in the neighborhood."

Misconception #2. Any arthritis can be seen on an MRI. Not true. If the arthritis is localized to one or more small areas, it can escape detection. This can be a source of frustration and anger in patients who undergo an outpatient knee procedure (arthroscopy) and are told after the surgery that they have arthritis. As far as they are concerned, the arthritis should have been detected preoperatively. The truth is that the possible existence of arthritis should indeed have been discussed preoperatively, but arthritis may not have been detectable on the MRI.

Misconception #3. If the arthritis looks bad on an x-ray, the person must be suffering quite a bit. Although patients with arthritis will eventually come to knee replacement surgery if they're young, heavy, and/or physically active, patients do not all develop pain at the same stage of arthritis. Why arthritis causes more pain in some people than in others remains one of the mysteries of the condition.

Misconception #4. If the arthritis looks bad on an x-ray, surgery is indicated. Yet again, not true. The following is a common ploy: The LK-SS surgeon demonstrates to the patient the "bad" arthritis on the x-ray and quickly gets the sucker, *er*, the patient to agree to surgery "before it's too late." This is very unscrupulous: First, as we have just noted, there is no correlation between how bad x-rays look and how a person might feel. Secondly, surgery should not be considered until reasonable nonoperative alternatives have failed. Finally, the arthritis pain may calm down on its own (see below). (Granted, some patients after an appropriate informed consent discussion may choose to bypass nonoperative measures and move right to surgery.)

The proper x-rays

Standard x-rays performed in an emergency room or by a health professional without a particular interest in knees will include a front and side view of your knee obtained while you lie on the x-ray table. If you have severe diffuse arthritis, these two simple views will suffice. The arthritis will be apparent and the diagnosis will be made. For arthritis that is more localized to one area or less advanced, however, these two views are likely to be inadequate.

To diagnose arthritis, at the very least you should be standing for the frontal x-ray, not lying down. This increases the odds that the narrowing of your joint will be apparent.

You should be getting an x-ray called the Merchant view, named after Alan Merchant, MD from California. This view, admittedly, takes extra time, added knowledge on the part of the person taking the x-ray, and some inexpensive, supplementary equipment. For this view, you lie on your back, legs bent over the end of the x-ray table, resting on a special device. This device keeps the knees bent at a specified angle, usually in the 30- to 45-degree range. With these x-rays, the doctor can determine if the kneecap is well seated in its groove (see Chapter 6). The doctor can also detect arthritis under the kneecap. In some patients, the kneecap is the *only* part of the knee to be arthritic, and without this view the arthritis may be completely missed!

There is at least one more view that should be obtained (the flexion PA view, a.k.a. Rosenberg, schuss, or standing flexion view), and it is discussed in Chapter 8.

Here is the bottom line: if you are sent for two x-rays of the knee—both taken lying down—and are then sent off for an MRI, chances are that you are dealing with an LK-SS. Someone is wasting your time and money.

There are exceptions. If you are under the age of forty, and it is very clear that the problem lies with the meniscus or one of the cruciate ligaments—neither of which show up on an x-ray—it is reasonable to skip the x-rays altogether and to go right for the MRI. Your insurance may force the doctor to obtain an x-ray first, and in this case, it is reasonable to obtain the two simplest views.

Are MRIs a waste of time?

No. As noted elsewhere in this book, there are multiple sources of knee pain some of which are best detected by an MRI. But in someone likely to have arthritis the answer is yes. If you are in your late sixties or older and you have had recurrent nagging knee pain, the chances are overwhelming that you have arthritis, even if you feel quite youthful. The above-mentioned x-rays will usually prove this. Even when these x-rays cannot demonstrate the arthritis, arthritis is still the most likely diagnosis.

Can an MRI be misleading?

You bet. Not only is an MRI not necessary in the context of arthritis, but it can be terribly misleading: anyone with arthritis is likely to have a reading of a torn meniscus on their MRI. In fact, to the radiologist, the torn meniscus may be more obvious than the arthritis, and the focus of the report may be on this alleged tear (See sample MRI report at the end of Chapter 2). This error in focus is a major concern because, as we saw in Chapter 2, the tear may or may not be real. Even if it is, the arthritis is by far the bigger problem. Imagine a house burning down. Does the fireman care whether there is a leaky faucet in the second floor bathroom?

Does he care whether the curtains in the living room are faded and need to be replaced? Of course not! The burning house takes precedence over everything else! Likewise, in a patient with chronic arthritic symptoms, just about *any* other condition detected by the MRI is likely to be trivial. In summary, the MRI in this setting muddies the waters.

Can pain come and go?

Not only can it come and go, but it typically comes and goes. The patient visiting the doctor with an arthritic flare-up will agree to just about anything, and the LK-SS doctor will take advantage of that by proposing surgery. At the other extreme, nonoperative remedies that allegedly require three months of continued use before they can be effective are taking advantage of the fact that, in that period of time, most arthritic flare-ups will have quieted down on their own.

Osteoarthritis versus Osteoporosis

The two words are similar and it stands to reason that they would describe similar conditions. Sorry, there is no connection between the two. Osteoarthritis is a condition of articular cartilage, more precisely the wearing out of this cartilage. Osteo*porosis* is a condition of bone, not cartilage; osteoporotic bone is relatively thin and fragile. Normal bone is to osteoporotic bone what dense fog is to light fog. Same stuff, less of it. One can have osteoarthritis with or without osteoporosis and vice versa.

The Treatment of Knee Arthritis

Nonoperative treatment

The Essentials:

- Rest. This may seem obvious, but people sometimes want to "work through" the pain. An arthritic flare-up demands rest. Gentle exercises can be resumed once the acute pain has abated.
- Heat and cold treatment. Although they are opposites, both heat and cold can be soothing. People generally like to be given specific formulas (for example, "do this for ten minutes, then do that for fifteen minutes"), but when it comes to heat and cold there is no right or wrong; it's a question of what works best for each individual person. I generally recommend ten minutes of one followed by ten minutes of the other. "Should the heat be moist or dry?" is a frequently asked question. Personally, I have not noted a difference, although individual patients will indicate a preference for one or the other. Beware of overdoing it! I've seen people burn themselves with a heating pad. Taking a sedative, drinking alcohol, and then falling asleep with an electric heating pad around your knee is not a good idea. When it comes to cold, the key is to not place ice directly on the skin. Believe it or not, you can get frostbite! Place a towel or wrap an elastic bandage between the ice and your skin. There are some commercially available neoprene wraps that house a gel pack that can be cooled or heated. In fact, two gel packs are a good idea

so that while one is being used the other can be either cooled or heated.

Medications

Oral medications (pills). These fall into many categories:

- Analgesics. These simply mask the pain. There is nothing wrong with that as long as you don't go out and abuse your arthritic joint while you're feeling better. These include acetaminophen (Tylenol®) and tramadol (Ultram®). Acetaminophen is an over-the-counter medication and is relatively safe. Nevertheless, it can have side serious effects that you don't even feel (e.g., liver damage), and you should inform your doctor if you find yourself taking this medication on a regular basis. (I feel that this is true for any medication or nutritional supplement.)
- Anti-inflammatories outside the steroid category are abbreviated NSAID for "non-steroidal anti-inflammatory drug." These calm the pain by chemically quieting the irritation associated with arthritis. Aspirin is the granddaddy of all NSAIDs. In ancient Greece women in labor were advised to chew on the leaves of the willow tree, as the salicin in the leaves would alleviate their pain. A salicin derivative has become the aspirin we know today. It is common wisdom that had it been discovered more recently, aspirin would never have been approved as an over-the-counter drug. It has multiple effects, it can interact with other medications, and it can adversely affect important biological functions for many weeks. For example, aspirin compromises platelets that help the blood to clot. This is very useful when aspirin is used as a blood thinner, but it is a major problem when blood thinning is contraindicated. You should definitely let your doctor know that you are taking aspirin when he or she prescribes *any other* medication.

Since the introduction of aspirin, dozens of NSAIDs have appeared and disappeared. Each new one naturally claims to be more powerful and have fewer side effects than existing NSAIDs. These side effects include stomach ulcers, which can hurt and cause serious bleeding, and more insidious damage to various organ systems such as the kidneys. The possibility has even been raised that NSAIDs can harm articular cartilage—the very root of the arthritis problem. I have not personally noted clinical evidence of this, but it is a point worth keeping in mind. A more recent class of NSAIDs is the so-called Cox-2 inhibitor [Celebrex® (celecoxib), Mobic® (meloxicam)] that is possibly even less likely to cause ulcers than naproxen (Aleve®) or ibuprofen (Advil®, Motrin®, or Nuprin®). This is a controversial topic. Note that the Cox-2 NSAIDs are *not better* pain relievers than the other NSAIDs. So if your current NSAID works and you are not at risk for ulcers (speak to your doctor about this), I would not switch (not to mention that Celebrex is more expensive).

The following is a common misconception: NSAIDs will reduce swelling. If the knee is swollen due to the irritation of arthritis, then yes, maybe. But if the swelling is the result of an injury, no! You might take ibuprofen, for instance, for the pain of a sprained ankle, but don't expect it to control that goose egg on the outside of your foot. NSAIDs control the pain of irritation but do not remove any water that has accumulated. The swelling from an injury will only resolve with rest, elevation, cold, compression, and tincture of time *[sic]*, powder of patience, and extract of expectation.

Keep in mind that patents run out after a few years. If you wonder why you don't hear of a great medication after a while, it's either because serious side effects have been discovered and the drug has been pulled off the market, or more likely, the patent has run out, and advertising is no longer cost effective. One medication that I have found to be effective is naproxen. It is convenient (twice-a-day dosage) and has been around for thirty-forty years. In its generic form it is relatively inexpensive, and you are not likely to wake up to the news that it has been pulled from the market. Remarkably, certain HMOs and insurance companies will not cover naproxen. They will, however, cover brand-only expensive NSAIDs. Go figure.

Did you know? You can combine an NSAID with an analgesic. For example, you can take naproxen with breakfast and dinner, and in between add acetaminophen. (Check with your doctor for your best dosage.)

Should you be asking for the very latest NSAID? By now, you know where I'm going with this. The obvious answer is the wrong one. New car models are usually better than the last one, but the same isn't true for medications or medical devices. Our government demands stringent tests, but there are still surprises. Remember Duract®? Of course not. It came out briefly in the late 1990s, and was history before you could say "complication." People got touchy about a few deaths here and there, and in the twitch of a liver enzyme, it was gone. Mind you, there may have been a little over-reaction on the part of the public. It really wasn't clear that the deaths were related to the medication, but the point remains that there can be surprises with new medications. Look up Vioxx®.

Then there are newer medications that aren't new at all. Take the case of the pain reliever Vicoprofen®. Vicoprofen consists of two separate medications put together: hydrocodone and ibuprofen. Hydrocodone is a strong, time-honored narcotic, and ibuprofen is a classic NSAID available as Motrin®, Advil®, Nuprin®, or, well, ibuprofen. These two medications are relatively inexpensive as generics.

Now here's the trick, so pay attention: although hydrocodone and ibuprofen are inexpensive on their own, one enterprising manufacturer combined the two medications to create the more expensive Vicoprofen! You'd have thought, "Nah, that'll never work." Who would pay a lot of money for a pill that consists of two inexpensive medications? Wrong again. This has been a popular medication. Did the doctors not recognize the ingredients? Did the drug company take unfair advantage of the confusion? No. For some people the convenience of swallowing one larger pill rather than two smaller pills is worth the extra expense. When it comes to you, you'll make your own decision about that.

And by the way, Vicoprofen® isn't alone. Many prescriptions and over-the-counter medications are pricey combinations of inexpensive products. Read the label and check with your pharmacist.

- Steroids. Steroids are a large class of medications. Steroids used for the pain of arthritis are different from anabolic steroids taken by some athletes. Cortisone was one of the original steroids, and the word "cortisone" is still used colloquially to denote any type of steroid. Steroids are strong anti-inflammatory medications, but they are associated with a long list of potential side effects when taken on a long-term basis. These include stomach ulcers, fluid retention, the raising of blood sugar, bone necrosis (bone strokes; see Chapter 7), and osteoporosis, to name but a few. Not everyone suffers from these side effects. The likelihood of developing one or more side effects depends on the dose of the medication and on the length of time the medication is taken. Despite their potential side effects, steroids are sometimes the only medications that will be effective, and doctors do still prescribe them. Interestingly, though the word cortisone is commonly used, it is no longer in orthopedic practice in the United States. Indeed, despite the fact that cortisone conjures up nasty things in people's minds, it is actually relatively weak. Prednisone, on the other hand, is much stronger and is a commonly prescribed steroid.
- Narcotics. An arthritic flare-up can be excruciating, and on a short-term basis, it is reasonable to take a narcotic. In the long run, it is not advisable for the reasons most of us know: they are addictive and they become less effective with time. (One is said to become *tolerant* to them.) Narcotics are constipating

and can make you drowsy. The most common narcotics—Percocet®, Percodan®, and Vicodin®—are combined with acetaminophen or aspirin. Check the label. If your narcotic already contains acetaminophen it is not a good idea to take even more acetaminophen without speaking to your doctor. The same goes for aspirin.

Consider this little-known fact: Pain medications work best when the knee *just* starts to hurt. It doesn't always pay to be a hero. When you feel the pain coming on, take something for it.

Injections

As unappealing as they are to most people, injections into the knee still have a place. These usually consist of a combination of a numbing agent (e.g. Novocain®) and a steroid. There are downsides to steroid injections: not only are they not curative, in the long run they may dry out the tissues and make them more prone to infection. There is therefore a limit to how many injections one can prescribe in a given period of time. This is a controversial topic; I limit steroid injections in the knee to three per year. Note that injections affect the site that has been injected and have limited impact on other body sites. If you've had three shoulder injections you can still receive a knee injection.

There exists a class of injections not related to steroids that was introduced in 1998. These are injections of a gooey material similar to the hyaluronic acid that your own knee makes (or should be making). Examples of this include, Orthovisc®, Suparz®, Euflexxa®, and Synvisc®. This is called viscosupplementation. The patient comes in for approximately three weekly shots. One product, SynviscOne®, combines all three injections into one. This minimizes the number of trips to the doctor but the extra volume is not always well tolerated by the patient. Injecting these products into the knee is akin to adding oil to a machine. The manufacturers have reported that these injections stimulate cartilage growth, but this has yet to be proven.

In my experience, these injections work best in patients whose arthritis is not advanced. They are pricey although usually covered by insurances. Overall, I've been pleasantly surprised by how well viscosupplementation injections work. The number of patients in my practice who've seen their knee replacement pushed back a few years is impressive. Critics would say we I'm witnessing the placebo effect at work (see Chapter 9), but based on the numbers, I don't think so. By the way, no, ultrasound is not needed to get a needle into the knee joint. The knee and shoulder are the two largest joints in the body for chrissake. The doctor does, however, have to use a needle long enough to make it through the "fat pad" at the front of the knee.

Nutritional supplements

The above-mentioned pills and injections do not cure arthritis; they simply quiet the pain. It would be very appealing to prescribe a medication that actually leads to the regeneration of worn-out cartilage. The manufacturers of two products—glucosamine and chondroitin sulfate—have made such a claim, and there is a school of thought that the two products should be taken together. Even the most fervent proponents recognize that the pain relief does not start until the products have been used regularly for at least one month. (Some say three months.) Since both products exist in the body, though not necessarily in that exact form, they cannot be called drugs. They are classified as nutritional supplements. The good news is that they are not under the control of the FDA and scientific validation is not required; they can be promoted and sold without having to wait the many years it takes for the FDA to determine that something is safe and effective. The bad news is that is that they are not under the control of the FDA and scientific validation is not required. They can be promoted and sold without having to wait the many years it takes for the FDA to determine that something is safe and effective! If the products are found to be ineffective, many people will have wasted an awful lot of money.

Fortunately, so far it appears that the products are safe. I do not know of side effects to these compounds. Anecdotally, a number of my patients swear by the product. Therefore, if money is not an issue (supplements can be expensive), I don't discourage my patients from trying them. But one has to keep in mind the fact that arthritic flare-ups quiet down on their own (see above), and that there can be placebo effects.

Know that as of this writing the American Academy of Orthopedic Surgeons has surveyed the medical literature and has not found convincing studies supporting the use of nutritional supplements for the prevention of arthritis nor convincing studies supporting steroid and viscosupplementation injections.

Diet

Rattlesnake meat, vinegar, honey, and white meat have all been touted as arthritis remedies, whereas tomatoes, eggplant, potatoes, sweets, and dairy products get the thumbs down. That is, if you believe in all this. I don't. It would be all too easy if a little rattlesnake and honey sandwich did the trick. Don't get me wrong: many of our scientific remedies come from natural products. If aspirin can come from the willow tree, then perhaps there is something medicinal about honey. But if this were the case, it would no longer be a secret, and right now if honey or vinegar is effective against arthritis, it's certainly a secret to me. "Sweetie, just a little extra vinegar on my salad and I'll join you on the tennis court!"

Physical Therapy (PT)

Physical therapy is a broad field including exercises and modalities (ultrasound, etc.) designed to promote motion and decrease pain. The exercises themselves can be divided into stretching and strengthening. When physical therapy is suggested to patients with arthritis, they occasionally have the mistaken impression that they are being sent for a strengthening program complete with pushing, pulling, huffing, and puffing. This is not appealing. However, PT in the setting of knee arthritis is more of the stretching, modality, and light strengthening variety.

An arthritic knee tends to get stiff; this is the body's natural response to arthritis. Moving an arthritic joint is what hurts. If the knee could be rendered completely stiff to the point where it didn't move at all, there would be no pain. Alas, there are problems with the body's attempt to freeze the joint: 1) The joint is never completely stiff, and so the pain persists; 2) A stiff joint doesn't work very well; 3) The stiffness is to some extent imparted by the chronic tensing of muscles, and this itself can contribute to pain. A portion of PT therefore involves restoring reasonable motion to the knee.

In addition to applying heat and cold, which patients can do on their own at home, PT can involve modalities such as ultrasound, and in more sophisticated settings, ionto- or phonophoresis. This is a process whereby drugs are applied to the skin and electrochemically led to diffuse through the skin. In my experience, these modalities tend to work better on knee problems that are relatively superficial (e.g., tendinitis) than on arthritis that lives down deep inside the joint. Nevertheless, it can be worth trying.

Massage. Tendons and muscles about the arthritic knee tend to be inflexible and sore. Massage aids in the stretching of these structures and thereby soothes the knee; it also soothes the soul. This is not an insignificant factor in the overall treatment of the patient whose pain has rendered him or her tense and irritable.

Taping. If the arthritis is confined to the kneecap and if the kneecap is poorly aligned, special taping techniques can be used to pull the kneecap toward its normal position (see the next chapter). This can take just enough pressure off the kneecap to afford some pain relief.

Arthritis and Exercise

Patients with knee arthritis tend not to exercise. Exercise hurts. There is also the fear that exercise will aggravate the arthritis.

Nevertheless, exercise is to be encouraged—not just for the sake of the knee but for the accepted cardiovascular benefits of aerobic exercise.

We are not talking about just any exercise. Jumping and twisting activities will tend to increase the pain. At the other extreme, water exercises are most helpful. The body is buoyant, and therefore by definition, less weight is placed across the knee when you're in water that's at least waist deep. Painful on land, running may be quite tolerable. It can be carried out in the shallow end of a pool, or with special flotation belts in the deep end. Likewise, kicking and jumping exercises are more readily performed in water. They strengthen the muscles, stretch the structures about the knee, contribute to cardiovascular fitness, and provide a sense of well-being. The water temperature should be comfortable, if not initially, at least within a few moments of exercising. If the water is too cold the muscles will become even more tense and painful.

For land exercises, cushioned shoes should be worn. Use of a treadmill is reasonable since the surface is relatively soft. The use of an exercise bicycle can address stiffness if the seat is high enough, but by and large, it is a neutral exercise: it won't help, and it won't hurt. Running is controversial. At one point, it was felt to cause arthritis, but recent studies suggest that in a normal knee, running does not promote arthritis. In a knee that is already arthritic, it may be a different story. I would tend to discourage running in someone who is quite bow-legged or knock-kneed.

Shoe wear

In a painfully arthritic knee, every jarring step hurts. Classic leather-soled shoes with hard rubber heels don't help the situation. Wearing shoes with softer heels such as running shoes, or inserting a cushioned insole can be of benefit. If you use an insole, make sure it is thick enough. Some foam insoles collapse like tissue paper and provide minimal cushioning. Silicone (not silicon) inserts are more durable and provide more cushioning.

Canes, sticks, and the like

Getting a patient to use a cane is a measure of how good a salesman the doctor is. Other than orthopedic shoes, no other treatment option has such a stigma attached to it. Where knee replacement surgery is high-tech, a cane just makes you look old—or so people feel. Naturally, men take to canes better than women. There are some very elegant canes, and men with canes can still conjure up a certain aura. A hiking stick may be more acceptable, though not necessarily when shopping down Fifth Avenue. Other alternatives include a golf umbrella or a shopping cart. No matter how you disguise it though, a cane is a hard sell. And yet, there is no question that using some kind of support will take pressure off the knee and provide some pain relief. A cane also addresses the unsteadiness some people feel as a result of their pain.

How to use a cane: if you've finally given in to using a cane, at least use it correctly. Most people use a cane that is far too long. There should just be a *little* bend in the elbow. You can't lean as effectively on a cane that's too long. Which hand? You may have heard that for hip problems the cane should be in the hand opposite the painful hip. This is correct. For knees, this is also true, though to a lesser extent.

Braces

Arthritis pain is partly the result of two bones rubbing. A snug brace or tightly wrapped elastic bandage can minimize such rubbing and assuage pain. That is the theory. In my experience, braces and wraps have a low probability of success—but not zero. With the use of tight wraps, there is the added concern that the blood circulation might be compromised. For patients whose arthritis is relatively mild and confined to just the inner aspect of the knee (medial arthritis), there are long-leg braces that imperceptibly push the knee into a less bow-legged and more knock-kneed position, thus taking pressure and pain off the inner aspect of the knee. In this specific situation, a brace can be safe and effective, especially if applied to a relatively thin muscular leg.

Acupuncture

The philosophy of acupuncture is based on the premise that human life flows along fourteen major meridians (channels). Each meridian governs a major organ system. Blockage of a meridian leads to pain or dysfunction while selective stimulation of meridians restores equilibrium and health. Acupuncture is an accepted adjunct to anesthesia, and I have occasionally seen patients obtain satisfactory relief from acupuncture in the setting of an arthritic knee. As with every other option listed, it is not a cure.

Surgery

When the time comes for surgery, you can see the glass as being half full or half empty: no one likes the idea of having surgery. On the other hand, where crutches, walkers, and wheelchairs were the only options available as recently as fifty years ago, today we live in an era where operations abound.

The best operation for you depends on a number of factors: How much of your knee is arthritic? Which part is arthritic? Are you particularly bow-legged or knock-kneed? Are you athletic? Are you on the younger side or older side? (Under sixty is younger here.) Are you willing to use crutches for three months?

Arthroscopy. This is an outpatient procedure where the surgeon inserts fine instruments through small puncture holes at the front of the knee (see Chapter 3). This allows the knee to be "cleaned out." Imagine a room that is dusty; the upholstery is worn down; plaster hangs off the ceiling. In this analogy, an arthroscopy cleans the furniture, freshens up the dangling plaster, and perhaps even rearranges the furniture a little. It doesn't re-upholster nor does it replaster. In other words, there is a limit to what an arthroscopy can do. As you may have gathered, the odds of arthroscopic success diminish with the size of the arthritic area(s). While "mechanical" symptoms such as painful clicking and catching improve the odds of success, by and large, an arthroscopic meniscectomy will not provide lasting benefits in the setting of an arthritic knee. Still, the younger the patient, the lower the threshold for trying a low-yield arthroscopy before moving on to a larger operation.

Osteotomy. If you live in the United States, chances are this operation won't be offered to you unless you are quite young. The operation involves cutting the bone and realigning the leg. In the most common scenario, a bow-legged knee is made knock-kneed. This is usually recommended to young people whose arthritis is confined to just the inner part of the knee. Crutches are commonly prescribed for three months. An osteotomy has disadvantages. It is somewhat difficult to predict who will obtain a good result. The osteotomy is a controlled fracture and sometimes doesn't heal, a situation requiring further surgery. Nerves and vessels can be injured during the operation. An osteotomy can make an eventual knee replacement more difficult and less successful. On the other hand, an osteotomy also has advantages: assuming all works out well, you can still participate in any sport you want and you can perform heavy labor.[5]

Total knee replacement. I never liked this term. It sounds awful. It conjures up the thought of someone taking out an entire knee. This is not the case. In knee replacement surgery, the worn-out ends of the bone are shaved off and replaced with metal and plastic on the other. An analogy can be made with capping a tooth or putting in fresh brake pads. A knee replacement should be called a knee resurfacing.

---

[5] If you have an academic interest in the subject, you may want to read the following article: Grelsamer RP, Unicompartmental Knee Arthritis—Current Concepts, *J Bone Joint Surg* 77A, no 2(1995): 278-292. Over 300 references are reviewed in this paper.

Knee replacements are like automobiles to the extent that they come in many models. They have basic similarities and certain differences. New models come out every year. Some have better track records than others. The major distinction between knee replacements and automobiles is that newer cars tend to be better than their predecessors whereas many if not most new knee replacements land on the trash heap. It's as big a misconception as there is in the world of orthopedic surgery. The public wants the latest implants without realizing what this implies. It means undergoing a knee replacement that is unlikely to stand the test of time! Without realizing it, the public is literally asking to be experimented on. If you want an implant that will last twenty years, you should ask for one that has been around that long.

Surgeons do not always recommend an implant based on its track record. They look for new and improved implants, convinced that the newest implants will solve the imperfections of existing implants. Unfortunately, the orthopedic highway is littered with implants that once held great promise—but then miserably failed. The failures occur years after the surgery. By then the manufacturers have moved on to the next great thing. Surgeons may not be swayed by manufacturers, being swayed instead by surgeons perceived to be leaders in the field. These leaders often have financial ties to the orthopedic manufacturers and for a price, are happy to promote new products. To its credit, the orthopedic community demands that speakers and authors reveal their financial ties to the orthopedic industry.

Partial knee replacements. In the orthopedic world, they are called unicompartmental knee replacements. These small implants replace only the part of the knee that is worn out, and are designed for patients whose arthritis is localized to just one part of the knee. Unicompartmental knee replacements are not terribly popular in the United States: they can be more difficult to implant than standard knee replacements, and because insurance companies erroneously see them as half a knee replacement, surgeons get reimbursed half of what they receive for a standard total knee replacement.

Unicompartmental knee replacements are much more popular in the rest of the world, and I suspect that they would be equally popular here if reimbursements here were different. I continue to believe that, in select patients, partial knee replacements are an excellent option.

A different type of partial knee replacement is the patellofemoral replacement that addresses arthritis around the kneecap. It shares many similarities with the unicompartmental replacement: the surgery is far less invasive than a total knee replacement, though the incision looks the same. You are far less likely to require a blood transfusion and you are left with all your ligaments and both of your menisci. Regaining motion is rarely an issue. The orthopedic literature of the last twenty years has been overwhelmingly positive—but the remaining two compartments of your knee have to be in pretty good shape for the procedure to be recommended (see Chapter 6).

Cartilage growing. This is a very exciting field. Cartilage normally doesn't grow in the human body. Once it is worn out or injured, it is gone forever. A more recent concept involves taking cartilage cells from patients, growing them in the laboratory, and reimplanting them in the patient. This is being tried with cautious optimism in young patients with localized loss of articular cartilage.

Molecular biology, genetic engineering, and stem cell implantation. The future of arthritis therapy lies in these areas. One day, people will view joint replacement surgery the way we quaintly look down upon the crude tools of yesteryear. The injection of that cell or this product will stimulate the body to create fresh cartilage in just the right place. Joint replacement surgeons will go the way of coopers and swordsmiths. For the moment, though, we all have to be grateful for the existence of knee replacements.

Arthritis Treatment

	Pros	Cons	Comments
Medication 1: Anti-inflammatories, including Advil®, Motrin®, Aleve®, Relafen®, Naprosyn®, Celebrex®, Vioxx®, etc. *Generic*: ibuprofen, naproxen	Take away pain without simply masking it	Can cause heartburn or ulcers. Possible cartilage damage in the long run.	Vary greatly in price
Medication 2: Acetaminophen Tylenol®	Few side effects in prescribed doses	Doesn't help solve the underlying problem	Inexpensive
Medication 3: Ultram®	Not an anti-inflammatory nor a narcotic	Can cause dizziness, slightly addictive	
Medication: Narcotic Tylenol® #3, Percocet®, Vicodin®, Norco®	Strong	Addiction, tolerance, drowsiness, constipation	For short-term use only
Physical Therapy	No side effects. Improves sense of well-being.	Time consuming. Variable effect.	
Injections 1: Steroids	No effects on stomach. Work within a week	Harm to tissues with *repeated* use	Not the same as taking "steroids" in the athletic sense
Injections 2: Hyaluran Orthovisc®, Synvisc®, Hyalgan®	"Natural." Rare side effects	Expensive. Repeated injections	Works best with mild arthritis
Heat and Cold	Soothing. No side effects.	Clumsy	Always keep a gel pack around the house
Brace / Support	Easy to use	Uncomfortable after a while	Borrow before buying

	Pros	Cons	Comments
Cane / Stick / Umbrella	Surprisingly effective	Yuk	You only look old if you act old
Cushioned shoes	Running shoes are fashionable	Running shoes aren't *that* fashionable	A cushioned insole helps too
Nutritional Supplements Glucosamine (Chondroitin Sulfate)	Harmless for most people	Take a long time to work. Felt to work better on animals!	Large variations in price for the same products
Acupuncture	No stomach side effects	Needles	Doesn't cure any more than the other treatments
Weight Control	Effective over time	No fun	This is about the only thing under your control!
Water Exercises	Stay fit without stressing the knee	Access can be difficult	
Surgery: Arthroscopy	Outpatient / Low risk	Limited benefit for advanced arthritis	A major surgical advance
Surgery: Osteotomy (leg realignment)	No metal or plastic inside the knee	Limited indications	Knock-kneed appearance after surgery.
Surgery: Cartilage growing	The only real cure for arthritis	Even more limited indications	Far from perfected. Stay tuned.
Surgery: Knee Replacement	Best chance for pain relief. Can be *total* or *partial* replacement.	Inpatient. Higher risk than arthroscopy.	Another surgical miracle of the twentieth century

	Pros	Cons	Comments
PRP (Platelet rich plasma) (of which there are different types)	Does no harm	Unproven	Not covered by insurance. Expensive.
Stem cells	Pending	Unproven (yet?). Harvesting requires anesthesia.	Even more expensive than PRP. Nascent technology

Dr. G's Ten Step Knee Arthritis Program

Like a man sitting among tin cans without a can opener, a person with knee arthritis can live miserably for lack of a step-by-step guide. Let me take you through a program that has worked well for my patients.

Step 1: Get the correct diagnosis. This sounds obvious, but not every painful or creaky knee is arthritic. If you are over sixty years old, chances are indeed that your knee pain is at least in part due to arthritis, but this is not automatic. If you are athletic, you may be suffering from the painful inflammation of one soft tissue or another. For example the tendon connecting your kneecap to the tibia (shinbone) may be inflamed, and this would be called tendinitis. After a few weeks of living with knee pain, see a health professional to obtain a specific diagnosis. Of course, as oft stated in this book, be leery of the MRI and be particularly leery of the torn cartilage diagnosis.

Step 2: Attitude adjustment. When given the diagnosis of arthritis, people not uncommonly go through mood swings, especially if they consider themselves to be too young to be tagged with this condition. Denial, anger, and depression are common. This is a natural reaction to receiving any bad news. Consider the following three case studies:

Fred is fifty-six and he'll be damned if he's going to modify his lifestyle. He's always jogged on the concrete track near his house and he regularly hikes the Appalachian Trail, which runs nearby.

Even if it means taking narcotics, he's not going to stop doing the things he loves.

Jane is forty-eight. She had the entire meniscus (cartilage) removed from her knee when she was a teenager and now she's been told of some early arthritis. She's bummed and feels sorry for herself. She cancels her tennis membership, takes out a subscription to *Modern Maturity*, and ponders her Last Will and Testament.

Arthur is fifty-eight. He's been an avid skier, a premier mogul smasher; regularly lifts weights at the gym. He's just been given the bad news about arthritis in his knee. Upon reflection he is grateful for the many years of thrilling skiing. Unlike Jane, he doesn't quit. He adapts. He still skis, but sticks to the easier runs; he uses the CADS device (cads.com) that pushes him up when he bends down. At the gym, he's given up the squats, the leg curls, and the "clean and jerks," and focuses more on the abdominals (abs) and the arms. He has signed up for water aerobics.

Clearly, Arthur has the right attitude. Fred is headed for trouble. When reality sinks in, he'll be that much more depressed. Jane is overreacting. She's letting the diagnosis of arthritis get to her and she's going to miss out on many enjoyable life experiences. She could still play tennis if she wanted to, but she should back off playing singles on hard courts. She could learn to enjoy doubles and could look into courts with more forgiving surfaces.

When receiving the diagnosis of knee arthritis, you must quickly realize that life is not over. You might need to make some adjustments, but there is no reason why you cannot enjoy life.

Step 3: Over-the-counter treatments. Early on, arthritis can be treated with simple remedies. For example, both heat and cold can be soothing—and they have no side effects. I strongly recommend this. Cushioned shoes, such as sneakers and running shoes, take the jarring out of each step. Even so-called city shoes occasionally come with rubber rather than leather soles. I also strongly recommend these. Acetaminophen, better known as Tylenol®, is a common, inexpensive analgesic which is certainly worth trying. Assuming that you have no stomach or kidney problems and are not taking a blood thinner, you can add an over-the-counter anti-inflammatory medication to your regimen. Many people obtain relief with naproxen or ibuprofen (available as generics or as the more expensive Aleve®, Advil®, Nuprin®, or Motrin®). Check with your doctor if you have any liver or kidney disease.

Step 4: Bracing. Wrapping something snuggly around the knee can provide relief. This can be in the form of an elastic wrap (Ace®, Coban®) or in the form of a knee support that is slipped on and adjusted with straps. This is also worth a try. Wear it as much or as little as you like.

Step 5: Exercise. The presence of knee arthritis does not spell the end of exercising. On the contrary. Arthritis tends to cause stiffness that in turn can lead to greater pain. The stretching and water exercises described in Chapter 11 are highly advised. In addition to conditioning your knee, these activities will provide you with a sense of well-being.

Step 6: Physical Therapy. A knowledgeable therapist can bring some life back to a painful, stiff knee. In addition to reviewing a stretching program with you, the therapist will provide you with massage and other modalities which, well, feel good. Because of the time and expense involved, start with Steps 1 to 5 before going to therapy.

Step 7: Prescription medications. Once you have been through Steps 1 to 4, you should discuss prescription medications with your doctor. These may have side effects, but they are stronger. My personal preference is for naproxen, the same medication that is listed in step 3. The prescription version is simply stronger. If you do not tolerate naproxen, many other similar medications are available.

Step 8: Use a hiking stick or an umbrella. Leaning on something when you walk takes pressure off the knee. If walking tends to worsen your pain, try a cane. Since canes have a stigma attached to them, consider using a big umbrella or a hiking stick. Some hiking sticks telescope down to a small size, a convenient travel feature.

Step 9: Injections. Injections provide relief on the order of days to months. I recommend alternating between steroid and viscosupplementation injections. (See Injection section above.)

Step 10: Surgery. When all else fails there is surgery. Fortunately there are many operations available, but keep in mind that there's no minor surgery, only minor surgeons.

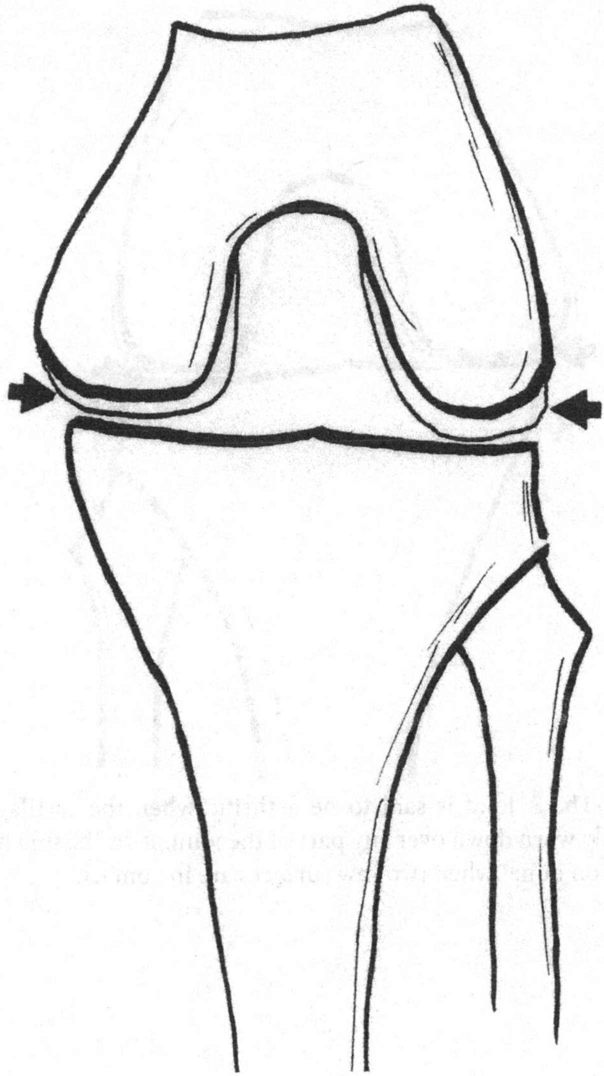

Figure 5-1a. The ends of bones are covered in a smooth, glistening white material that is six times smoother than ice. This is called articular cartilage (solid arrows).

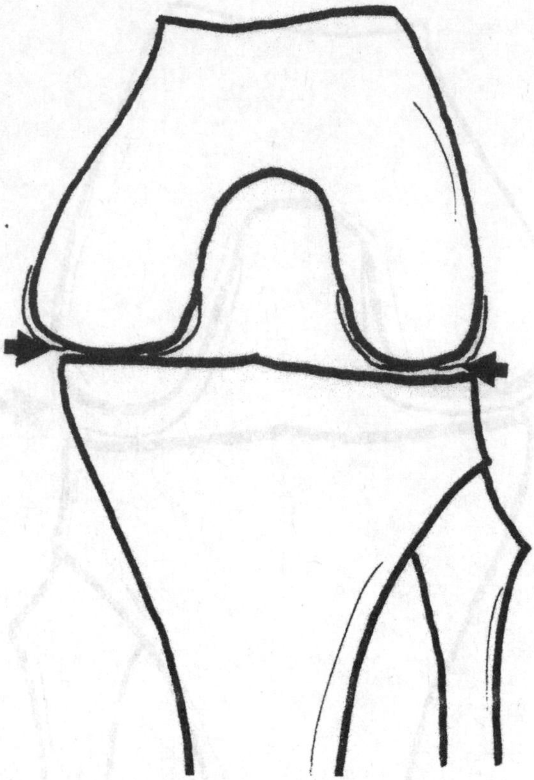

Figure 5-1b. A joint is said to be arthritic when the cartilage has completely worn down over any part of the joint. It's a "kissing lesion" or "bone on bone" when two raw surfaces are in contact.

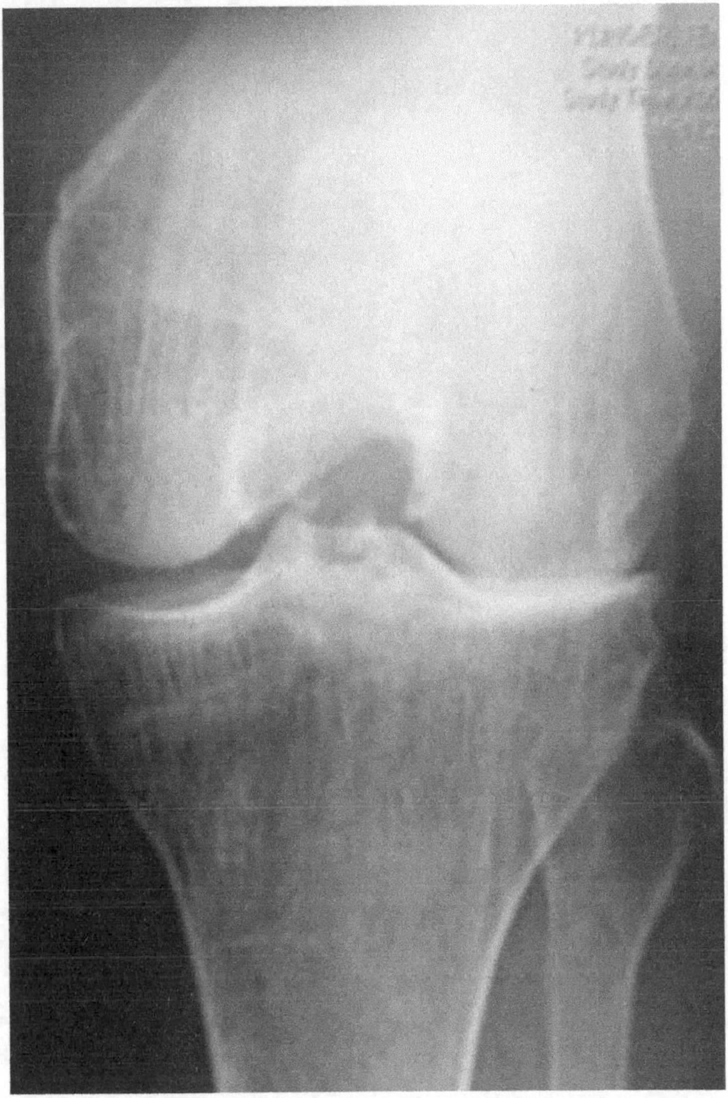

Figure 5-2. On the right side of the x-ray the two bones are touching; the cartilage lining both the femur and tibia is worn out. A classic arthritic picture—taken with the patient standing and knees bent (see Chapter 8).

CHAPTER 6

The Hidden Causes of Knee Pain: Part I—Your Kneecap: Chondromalacia, Patellofemoral Syndrome

Summary Soundbite:

- Kneecap issues are often misdiagnosed and over operated.

If you rise awkwardly from a kneeling position, feel a pop, and tear a meniscus cartilage in your knee, the diagnosis will be obvious to any orthopedic practitioner. Not all conditions are so clear. Somewhere between the obvious and the unsolvable lie well-described conditions that elude the average knee care provider. These I term the hidden causes of knee pain.

What's wrong with this picture?

Sally M. is thirty-four years old. She was fine until she fell and landed on her left knee four years ago. She underwent an MRI within a week of the injury and was told she had a torn cartilage. Physical therapy was next consisting of an exercise bicycle and "funny pads" placed around her knee. Six weeks after her injury, she underwent an arthroscopy; she was told that she'd had a torn meniscus and that the knee had been cleaned up. Yet she felt no better. She went for more sessions of exercise on the bicycle until her insurance refused to pay for more therapy. Various anti-inflammatory medications were tried, and she dipped her toes into the world of narcotics. Her friends and employer started to see a ploy for sympathy. There was a psychological evaluation. Another orthopedist recommended another MRI and a second arthroscopy to remove scar tissue from the first operation.

The above scenario is more common than you might imagine. There are many things wrong with this picture, some of which you probably recognize from reading the previous chapters.

1. The MRI soon after the simple injury was not reasonable: it was not likely to affect the treatment in a positive way, and indeed it misled both the surgeon and the patient.
2. The finding of a torn cartilage in someone who has bumped his or her knee is likely to be either wrong or irrelevant.
3. Surgery for a torn cartilage in this setting was doomed to failure right from the start.
4. Simply using an exercise bicycle, putting weights on your ankle, and getting a little electrical stimulation is simply not adequate physical therapy for a number of knee conditions.
5. The doctors made no realistic attempt to find the true cause of Sally's pain.

Pain at the front of the knee has many potential sources, some of which are not even in the knee. A number of these conditions will not be detected on an MRI—a test that doctors rely on excessively. As doctors squeeze more and more patients into their schedule, it is increasingly the MRI that makes the diagnosis. The doctor listens to you for a few seconds, puts his hands on your knee for a few moments, and then waits for the MRI report to inform you of your diagnosis. By this point in the book, we've discussed at length why that approach is problematic.

Anterior Knee Pain, a.k.a. Chondromalacia, a.k.a. Patellofemoral Syndrome

These are all synonyms.

They all refer to pain at the front of the knee that your doctor can't quite figure out. Anterior knee pain simply means that you have pain at the front of the knee; presumably you know this already.

Chondromalacia is Latin for "soft cartilage." For much of the last century, it was felt that pain at the front of the knee was the result of excessively soft cartilage. We now know this is not so; moreover, the word "chondromalacia" has come to take on multiple meanings: Pain in the front of the knee, pain from an improperly positioned kneecap, cartilage damage under the kneecap, arthritis under the kneecap, cartilage damage or arthritis anywhere in the knee, and perhaps most commonly, "I don't know what's wrong with you." Over the last fifty years, chondromalacia has become an accepted expression, and in the United States, there is even an insurance code for it. If your pain lies toward the front of the knee and the doctor can't find much wrong, he will in all likelihood tell you that you are suffering from chondromalacia.

Due to its multiple meanings, however, it has become a source of confusion and miscommunication. Gradually, the term is being abandoned, though not fast enough.[6] I continue to feel that the word should be abandoned altogether.

Patellofemoral syndrome is orthopedic double-talk pure and simple. A syndrome in the world of medicine is a specific set of patient complaints combined with specific findings on the physical examination and/or specific test results.

No such specific set of signs, symptoms, and test results exists in people suffering from pain at the front of their knee.

---

[6] RP Grelsamer, G Moss, G Ee, and S Donell, The patellofemoral syndrome; the same problem as the Loch Ness Monster?, *The Knee* 16, no 5, (2009): 301–302.

Patellofemoral syndrome has simply replaced chondromalacia in certain medical offices and also means "I do not know what is wrong with you."

Your Kneecap

Basic Anatomy

The kneecap (patella) is the small, round bone in front of the knee. It is a complex lever that provides a mechanical advantage to the thigh muscles. Without a kneecap, your quadriceps muscles at the front of the thigh would work harder.

As the knee bends and straightens, the kneecap glides in a groove (the trochlea or trochlear groove located at the end of the thighbone). Roughly speaking, the undersurface of the kneecap looks like a broad "U" and it matches the "U" shape of the groove. This presents a number of potential problems: the fit can be too loose causing the kneecap to slip in and out and leading to a sensation of giving way (See Figures 6-1 and 6-5). In other patients the kneecap can be poorly positioned (malaligned) within the groove—much as the wheel on a car might be out of alignment. It can be painful when one side of the kneecap gets overworked.

On occasion, the groove is shallow or flat or even inverted. In other words, it is possible for the groove to be convex like a fried egg, in which case the kneecap/trochlea construct is highly unstable.

There are four muscles connected to the upper part of the kneecap, and collectively these are called the quadriceps (literally "four heads"). These include the rectus femoris, the vastus intermedius, the vastus lateralis, and the vastus medialis.

All tend to pull the kneecap toward the head, but whereas the first two pull straight up, the vastus lateralis pulls the kneecap up and out, so to speak, and the vastus medialis pulls up and in (see Figure 6-2). The kneecap is connected to the "quads" via a broad, flat tendon called the quadriceps tendon. At its other end, the kneecap is attached to the tibia by way of the patellar tendon, occasionally called the patellar ligament.[7] The net result of all these connections is a straightening of the knee when the quadriceps muscles contract.

In more ways than one, the kneecap mechanism ("extensor mechanism") rounds a corner. Not only is the kneecap draped over the end of the thighbone like a waterfall, but when seen from the front, the quadriceps, kneecap, and patellar tendon also form an angle (see Figure 6-3). This angle (called the quadriceps or Q angle) causes the kneecap to be pulled toward the outside part of the knee every time the quadriceps muscles contract; this is termed the bowstring effect. In some people, the Q angle is particularly pronounced and represents a form of kneecap malalignment.

The outside (lateral) wall of the trochlear groove is higher than the inside (medial) wall. This counters the bowstring effect, keeping the kneecap within its groove.

There are other parts of the anatomy that either exacerbate or counter the bowstring effect. For example, the lateral retinaculum is a tough, broad band of tissue attached to the entire outside (lateral) part of the kneecap.[8] Predictably, it tends to pull the kneecap to the outside and it increases the bowstring effect. On the inside (medial) aspect of the kneecap lies the medial retinaculum. It tends to be weaker than its lateral counterpart and receives significant assistance from a muscle called the vastus medialis obliquus (VMO). The VMO is actually the lower portion of the vastus medialis that we discussed above. People with malalignment of their kneecap (see below) are commonly cursed with a VMO that is deficient: the

[7] Bands of tissue connecting one bone to another are called ligaments while bands of tissue connecting muscles to bone are called tendons. Since the biological rope we are discussing connects the kneecap to the shinbone, in one sense, it is a ligament. On the other hand, functionally speaking, this rope is but a continuation of the quadriceps muscles (and of the quadriceps tendon). In this sense, our rope is a tendon; thus the term patellar tendon.

[8] Lateral means away from the midline; medial means toward the midline. Thus the little toe is lateral to the big toe and the big toe is medial to the second toe.

fibers are too vertical and they don't attach themselves far enough down on the kneecap. The consequence of this suboptimal setup is a VMO that does not adequately balance the bowstring effect. This allows the kneecap to be pushed up against the lateral wall of the trochlea or to be pushed out of the trochlea altogether.

In cross section, the kneecap looks like a triangle with rounded sides. It lies flat in the trochlea. In other words, relative to the horizon it is not tilted. (It sits like a hat on your head, not a beret off to the side.)

Perhaps you think of the kneecap as just being a bone; in fact, its undersurface features the thickest and softest cartilage in the human body. (If you are biomechanically inclined, know that it is also the most permeable to joint fluid.)

What could possibly go wrong?

Kneecap Malalignment

In my experience, this represents a great area of misdiagnosis about the knee. It is a field that is very poorly appreciated by orthopedists, physical therapists, rheumatologists, radiologists, physiatrists (rehabilitation specialists), chiropractors, and other health professionals dealing with knee pain.

By and large, kneecap problems are underdiagnosed and over operated.

If your knee slips out of its groove, there is a reasonable chance that the correct diagnosis will be made—and even so, many an unstable kneecap has been mistaken for a torn ACL. If, however, your knee simply hurts because of malalignment, chances are that the person looking after you will misdiagnose it.

Considering the number of excellent doctors around and considering how common kneecap problems are, you probably wonder how it could be possible for the condition to be so frequently misdiagnosed. The answer lies in the erratic dissemination of medical knowledge. A new concept or treatment may occasionally sweep over the medical community (e.g., Viagra®), but more commonly it gradually seeps into everyday practice, a little faster here, a little slower there. Kneecap conditions are well recognized in certain parts of the world and more poorly acknowledged in others. Strange as it may seem, kneecap conditions are still relatively unappreciated in the United States.

Kneecap issues mimic other conditions about the knee. In 1940, Dr. Karlsson in Sweden noted that surgeons were commonly taking out torn cartilage for what was really a kneecap problem—and this was in 1940 when taking out a cartilage was a serious endeavor (a large scar and five days in the hospital). Nowadays, removing a meniscus is a relatively small outpatient procedure that neither doctors nor patients think twice about. The problem of "mistaken identity" has therefore been hugely magnified! Europeans are not the only ones who have picked up on the problem: Jack Hughston, a famous orthopedist from our very own country, noted as far back as 1960 that "the orthopedic surgeon who has not mistaken a recurrent subluxation of the patella for a torn medial meniscus has undoubtedly had a very limited and fortunate experience with knees and meniscectomies." And yet the message has been painfully slow to get through to the rank and file. A large percentage of patients with knee pain get a (needless) MRI (erroneously read as showing a torn cartilage, of course), and a large percentage of these patients are scheduled for unnecessary surgery.

In the United States, orthopedists are rarely rescued by radiologists. Radiologists detect fractures, arthritis, and various bone diseases that the orthopedist might not have suspected; but when it comes to the kneecap, the radiologist is likely to know even less than the orthopedist. Even when an abnormality exists with regard to the patella, the x-ray report is likely to simply read "no fracture, no dislocation." This is technically correct: there is no fracture and crudely speaking, everything appears in place. But the fact that the kneecap might by lying too high, too far to the right or left, or in a tilted position is often altogether omitted.

The simplest views of the knee are called the AP (anteroposterior) and the lateral. The AP is the front-to-back view, the lateral is the side view. If the lateral is carried out just right, a great deal of information can be obtained with regard to the kneecap and its underlying groove. An additional view called the Merchant view provides yet further information. For this view, you lie on your back with your legs off the x-ray table resting on a special device which maintains your knees bent anywhere from 30 degrees (ideally) to 45 degrees (see Chapter 8). This view should be obtained in just about anyone with knee pain.

The perfect crime

The kneecap can lie in a tilted position, lateral side down (Figure 6-4). This is most commonly associated with an excessively tight lateral retinaculum, and in my experience, is the most common form of kneecap malalignment.

If the doctor palpates the undersurface of the patella by curling his fingers around its lateral border, this is normally painless. This maneuver on the other hand can be painful in patients whose kneecap is chronically tilted.[9]

The combination of tilt and tenderness is, in my opinion, evidence that part of your problem is coming from the kneecap.

Know that this is not a universal truth. Otherwise knowledgeable health professionals state that tilted kneecaps are normal, and they base that argument on the fact that they often see tilted kneecaps that are painless. It is my feeling that they are confusing the term "normal" in the everyday sense of the term with "normal" as used in the world of medicine. "Normal" in everyday language means common or acceptable. In that sense, it is indeed "normal" for a segment of the population to develop cancer or heart disease. But a medically normal condition is one that does not lead to death, disease, or pain, and in that sense of the word, cancer and heart disease are clearly not normal. Kneecap malalignment

[9] Cartilage itself has no nerve fibers and cannot register pain. The lateral retinaculum and the underlying patellar bone, however, are richly innervated and very sensitive to pain.

is normal in the common sense of the word, but not in the medical sense. An analogy can be made with flat feet: they are common and not necessarily painful, but they are not normal.

The innocent patient presents to the doctor with knee pain. Using a misleading MRI (see Chapter 2) the surgeon sells an operation to the patient. The surgeon informs the patient that it may take a few weeks for the full effects of the surgery to be apparent. (This is actually true.) Following surgery, the patient receives physical therapy and does eventually get better. The surgeon has earned a few dollars, the patient is thrilled with her surgeon, everybody's happy, and there's no problem, right?

Wrong.

You've just witnessed the perfect crime. With time and appropriate physical therapy, the patient was going to get better anyway! Who is ever going to know? This is a victimless crime. These useless operations lead to high insurance premiums, but who is going to notice? There is another catch though: There is no risk-free surgery. Even with a minor procedure such as an arthroscopy, some patients develop complications. This then is my main objection to gratuitous knee surgery.

Making the right diagnosis

One of the first things they teach you in medical school is that you can't make a diagnosis you haven't thought of. Therefore, the right diagnosis will never be made if the doctor isn't at least considering your kneecap as a potential problem. The diagnosis of a kneecap that doesn't sit or track properly is made on the physical examination and can often be confirmed on routine x-rays or an MRI. Therein lies another problem: the doctor has to actually take the time to examine you thoroughly. If he wants to confirm the diagnosis on an x-ray, he has to be particularly adept at ordering and reading those special views. Should he wish confirmation on an MRI, the doctor has to make sure that the MRI is complete (see Chapter 2) and that either he or the radiologist is familiar with the interpretation of kneecap problems on MRIs. In my experience, these conditions are not always met.

Treatment

The kneecap cure

While making the diagnosis can be difficult, the treatment for a kneecap that doesn't sit or track properly is surprisingly straightforward (see Table 1). Ninety-five percent of patients improve with a nonoperative program the cornerstone of which is appropriate physical therapy. The key word here is appropriate. Twenty minutes on an exercise bicycle, a few warm towels, and electrical stimulation with those funny little pads do not constitute an appropriate program for this condition. It is upsetting to find people scheduled for surgery on the basis of failed physical therapy when in fact they never had suitable therapy to begin with.

Therapy for this condition includes stretching of the major muscle groups about the knee. This includes the hamstrings at the back of your thigh, the quadriceps muscles at the front of your thigh, the adductor muscles at the inner thigh, and the iliotibial band that runs along the outer part of the thigh. You can perform some of these exercises at home (see Figure 11-6). In fact, you should. It's like learning the piano: practice between the lessons! Through skillful manipulation, the therapist can also gradually stretch the lateral retinaculum (see Basic Anatomy above).

Taping is a technique whereby special tape is applied to the front of the knee. It is applied in such a way as to pull the skin in one direction or another. Because the kneecap is (loosely) connected to the skin, the kneecap is pulled along the direction of the skin. Thus taping pulls the kneecap toward a more normal position. This at least is the theory. The extent to which this really takes place remains a subject of controversy. But the fact that a number of patients are helped by this approach is, in my experience, unequivocal. Some people learn the technique from their therapist and tape their knee at home. Biofeedback and surface electromyography are more sophisticated (less accessible) physical therapy modalities that help the patient monitor progress. Most important of all, physical therapy for kneecap conditions requires significant attention on the part of the therapy team. Not all therapy outfits are geared to that approach, and unfortunately, in a managed care setting it is true that this kind of attention may not be cost effective for the therapist.

Your core control of the kneecap begins with the pelvic, abdominal, and buttocks muscles. An expert therapist will evaluate, stretch, and strengthen those areas as needed.

Surgery

In case you've zoomed right to this section, keep in mind that it is the rare patient with kneecap problems who needs surgery. If you need surgery, it's either because you've failed a thorough nonoperative program, your malalignment is truly severe, or your kneecap is very arthritic.

Compared to surgery for other conditions, surgery for kneecap problems is less rewarding, and choosing the right operation is a major source of debate at orthopedic meetings. Over 150 procedures have been described through the years, and there are currently dozens of procedures still in use. There are two camps: the first includes surgeons who perform an outpatient (small incision) procedure first and then come back later for a bigger procedure if necessary. The second includes surgeons who perform the definitive procedure from the start if they feel that the small procedure has a low chance of success. By and large I have been in the second camp. Patients are not usually grateful for an operation that doesn't work, even if it is a small operation. They are even less grateful when they discover that the small operation isn't always so small when it comes to recovery and complications. In select cases, however, I am amenable to first trying the smaller procedure.

For patients whose kneecap slips in and out of the groove, the challenge for the surgeon is to tighten the kneecap without tightening it so much that arthritis will develop in later years. At least one operation has become notorious for this complication.[10] In patients whose main complaint is pain, the challenge is simply to provide lasting pain relief.

Kneecap operations can be divided into those that realign the kneecap and those that do not. Realignment operations are, by and large, performed when the kneecap is felt to be out of place. These operations can also be performed if the cartilage under the kneecap is unhealthy, and if the surgeon feels that moving the kneecap one way or the other will take pressure off these unhealthy areas.

The orthopedic community distinguishes between proximal and distal realignment operations. The word "proximal" means close to the center of the body; "distal" means far. Thus, in orthopedic lingo, the ankle would be distal to the knee, the hip would be proximal to the knee, and so forth. Proximal procedures involve surgery on the tissues that surround the kneecap while distal realignments are performed further down on the tibial tuberosity—the bump at the top of the tibia (shinbone) where the kneecap ligament attaches itself (see Figure 6-6).

The following is a thumbnail summary of some the operations you're likely to hear about.

Proximal realignments include:

The lateral retinacular release (commonly referred to as lateral release): when the lateral retinaculum is tight, it tugs on the kneecap. The kneecap becomes tilted like a beret and/or pulled off to the side. The concept of the lateral release is therefore simple. As described in the 1970s by Ficat in France and by Merchant in the United States, the lateral retinaculum is cut as it inserts onto the kneecap and the

[10] The Hauser procedure that was developed in the 1930s by Emil Hauser from Chicago.

patellar tendon. It was a brilliant idea that was rapidly embraced by the orthopedic community. The concept of an unstable kneecap has been as ancient as human civilization, but until the 1970s no one had thought that a *tilted* kneecap could be painful. The fact that a relatively simple procedure could cure this heretofore mysterious kneecap pain made the operation deliciously enticing. The procedure became that much more appealing in the 1980s when it was discovered that the release could be carried out via a small incision or even arthroscopically (without incisions or scars): the surgeon visualizes the inside of the knee through an arthroscope.[11] He or she then cuts the lateral retinaculum from the inside of the knee, proceeding up to—but not through—the skin (there are variations on this). The lateral release became wildly popular, and surgeons began to expand the indications for this procedure to anybody with unexplained knee pain. It was too good to be true.

And it was. Results started to come in. In the first place, the lateral release is not completely innocuous. Coursing through the lateral retinaculum are a group of blood vessels that readily bleed when cut. These are the "geniculate" vessels. They are pernicious to the extent that, when cut, they may not bleed right away. Instead they go into spasm. This stops the bleeding; at least temporarily. Within a short time—but *after* the patient has left the operating room—the spasm resolves. The geniculates begin to bleed. The knee swells as it fills with blood. This is painful and limits the patient's knee motion. At the first post operative visit the surgeon has to "tap" the knee, that is, place a needle into the joint to draw out the blood. This is not a major crowd pleaser. Moreover, even though the lateral release leaves little to no traces, it is still an operation. It is therefore subject to all the potential complications of an operation. These include infections and RSD (see Chapter 7), complications that are rare. Less rare is the very real complication of not making the patient feel any better.

---

[11] The arthroscope is a pencil-like instrument introduced into a joint via a small hole (see Chapter 3).

There are a number of reasons why a lateral release by itself may not work: the extent of the release may be insufficient; it can be excessive with the kneecap now slipping too far in the opposite direction. It does not predictably correct all that is wrong: as part of the overall problem, the medial retinaculum might be lax and the VMO muscle can be deficient. The Q angle is occasionally elevated, and arthritic lesions may be present under the kneecap or in the trochlea. The kneecap can lie too high (patella alta) or too low (patella baja, a.k.a. infera). The trochlea can be convex instead of being concave. With the exception of very specific arthritic lesions, the lateral release is not going to address these deficiencies.

At the present, the role of the isolated lateral release is a hotly contested issue in the world of orthopedics.

The medial plication / VMO advancement.

The medial retinaculum can be lax and the VMO can be flimsy and poorly positioned. To address this, the medial retinaculum is detached from the kneecap and then reattached over the kneecap. Alternatively, a portion of the retinaculum is removed, and the remainder is reattached to the side of the kneecap from whence it came. Either way, the kneecap is pulled medially (toward the inside). The VMO can be detached from the quadriceps tendon and from the upper medial corner of the kneecap and pulled down in the direction of its fibers onto the kneecap. Again, the effect is to pull the kneecap over medially.[12] This operation is usually performed in combination with a lateral release and therefore requires a separate incision. The alternative is an incision down the middle of the knee that gives the surgeon access to both sides of the kneecap.

Distal realignments include:

a. The Elmslie-Trillat moves the tibial tuberosity medially (to the inside) (Figure 6-7). It cannot be used in children with

[12] And posteriorly (toward the back) if overdone.

much growth left, as it can harm part of the growth plate at the top of the shinbone.

Because an abnormal position of the tibial tuberosity leads to an elevated Q angle (see above), the least controversial indication for the Elmslie-Trillat operation is an elevated Q angle. The most controversial aspect of the operation is its use in patients whose tibial tuberosity is normally positioned to begin with.

When the tibial tuberosity is moved to its new position, it needs to be fixed with one or two screws, and the patient has to limit his or her activities for six to twelve weeks until the tuberosity has healed in its new position. Depending on how solidly fixed these screws are, a cast or soft knee immobilizer will be used until the tuberosity has sufficiently healed.

b. The Maquet: This operation is named after the Belgian surgeon who first described it. It has lost much of its popularity, but it remains an accepted procedure. It is designed to lift the kneecap out of the trochlear groove, thus taking pressure off it. Unfortunately, it mostly lifts the nose (distal pole) of the kneecap and does not predictably relieve pain. To carry out the operation, the tibial tuberosity is partially split off from the underlying shinbone, and a piece of bone is inserted between the shinbone and the tuberosity (Figure 6-7). This elevates the tuberosity, which in turn elevates the patellar tendon, which in turn elevates the tip of the kneecap.

Just how much to elevate the tuberosity, where the bone should come from, what bone substitutes are acceptable, how the tuberosity should be stabilized until it heals (screws?), and the indications for the operation are just some of the controversies surrounding it.

c. The Fulkerson (AMZ): This is a combination of the two tibial tuberosity transfers described above and has essentially supplanted them. The tuberosity is both elevated and transposed medially (to the inside) through a single oblique cut between the tuberosity and the underlying bone. John Fulkerson, MD, has popularized it in the United States, and most orthopedists refer to the procedure as the Fulkerson.

Dr. Fulkerson himself has called the procedure the AMZ for anteromedialization. It combines the advantages and disadvantages of the Elmslie-Trillat and of the Maquet. My personal indication for this operation is a patient who in my opinion would benefit from both the Elmslie-Trillat and the Maquet (see Figure 6-7).

d. The distal transfer: If the kneecap sits too high in the groove (patella alta), the tibial tuberosity can be brought distally (down toward the foot) by a fraction of an inch. This is less commonly performed in the United States than the above-mentioned operations. It is in part because severe patella alta is relatively uncommon and partly because patella alta is under-recognized (see Chapters 2 and 8).

It is important to note that distal realignments can be performed in combination with any of the proximal realignments. This makes for an impressive number of surgical permutations. The knowledgeable surgeon will think this through carefully and do his/her best to put together the combination that's right for you.

Denervation. By cutting through both the medial and lateral retinaculum, the surgeon interrupts a significant percentage of the nerves that transmit pain from the kneecap. Cynics will say that the above-mentioned operations relieve pain not because the kneecap has been realigned but because the sensory nerve supply has been interrupted. There may be some truth to this; but not enough truth to make it a completely reliable approach.

Kneecap Arthritis

Sometimes, putting the kneecap where it belongs is not enough. If arthritis already exists under the kneecap or in the underlying trochlear groove, one can still have pain even if the kneecap is correctly positioned. Assuming you've tried and failed the arthritis treatment choices listed in Chapter 5, the surgeon now has the following options: He or she can move the kneecap up, down, left, or right in such a way as to take pressure off the raw area(s). The larger the arthritic area, the less this approach is likely to work.

The raw surfaces can be carefully drilled or hammered with a sharp pointy object in order to create small holes through the hard underlying bone. This brings blood to the surface and with it, hopefully, cartilage-producing cells. This is not a predictable technique, but it is relatively void of complications. In its various incarnations, the operation has been called the Pridie technique and is currently referred to as the microfracture technique.

Other options include taking cartilage plugs from a different part of the knee to replace the worn area—the OATS procedure (similar to the hair plug technique). Alternatively, a very small amount of cartilage can be harvested from another part of the knee; sent to a laboratory which cultures the cartilage until it has grown to the size of a thimble; reintroduced into the knee, and placed into the raw, arthritic areas. This is called autologous chondrocyte implantation (ACI).

One company markets juvenile cartilage cells imbedded in a gel that is placed in the cartilage defect. In the future, stem cells will be imbedded in the gel, the cells will differentiate into cartilage cells which in turn will produce normal articular cartilage.

The worn undersurface of the kneecap can be replaced with a plastic implant while the trochlear groove is covered with a fine metallic shield. This is, in effect, a *partial* knee replacement—with many of the pros and cons associated with joint replacement surgery (see Chapter 5). I have had good results with this approach. A *complete* knee replacement is always an option, as it is for any arthritis anywhere in the knee.

As a final choice, the kneecap can be removed outright. This is called a patellectomy. Although some patients can obtain pain relief, the kneecap serves a useful function as we saw at the top of this chapter, and as of this writing, there is no easy turning back once the kneecap has been removed. The operation is not sufficiently predictable with regard to pain relief, especially if arthritis is also present in the trochlear groove. Tumors and infection are the primary indications for a patellectomy.

Table 1. The nonoperative treatment of patellar pain.

Treatment	Pros	Cons
Activity Modification	Works to some extent	Are you willing to give up that sport?
Physical Therapy	Usually helps	Needs to be supervised by a very knowledgeable person
Home Exercises	Effective in maintaining what's been taught in physical therapy	Boring
Brace	Few side effects	Trial and error to find the right one.
Anti-inflammatory Medication	Quiets pain by diminishing inflammation	Can't take pills forever
Analgesic (e.g. acetaminophen)	Few stomach side effects	Limited effect
Cold / Heat	Quiets pain without pills	Mainly useful at home Cumbersome
Injections	Work in the short run	Limited effect Who wants injections?
Weight Reduction	Takes a great deal of pressure off the kneecap	Takes a great deal of self-discipline

Incomplete Imaging
525 Main Street
Anywhere, USA

John Smith, MD
Anywhere, United States of America

Patient: Mary Smith
Study: MRI Left Knee

Images were obtained in the sagittal plane using a T1 weighted pulse and T2 weighted pulse sequences. Coronal T1 weighted images were also obtained.
Osseous structures are grossly intact.
The anterior and posterior cruciate ligaments are preserved. A Grade I signal is noted in the medial collateral ligament (MCL).
The extensor mechanism is intact.
A Grade II tear is found in the posterior horn of the medial meniscus without extension to the surface. The lateral meniscus is normal.
A small suprapatellar joint effusion is noted. There is a Baker's cyst.

IMPRESSION:

Grade II tear of the posterior horn of the medial meniscus
Grade I tear of the MCL
Joint effusion
Baker's cyst

The above shows a misleading MRI report in a patient with kneecap pain. Note the inaccurate or irrelevant findings. I count at least five of them.

1. The so-called Grade II tear of the meniscus is not a tear. It represents a chemical change within the meniscus (cartilage), it is not visible to the naked eye, and it does not cause knee pain.
2. An injury is required to tear the medial collateral ligament (MCL). This patient had no injury. The "Grade I" tear seen

by the radiologist therefore represents a slight variation in the composition of the ligament, and does not shed light on the patient's condition.

3. Joint effusion indicates water on the knee. This is found in just about any patient whose knee is irritated for whatever reason. In and of itself, it is not painful, and its presence does not help the doctor diagnose the source of the pain.
4. The Baker's cyst is a pouch at the back of the knee. Normal joint fluid sometimes collects in that pouch. It is a common finding and is not painful.
5. The radiologist proceeds to omit the most glaring problem: the patient has a serious disorder of the kneecap and of the underlying groove. The reason for the omission is simple: the MRI is incomplete. Note in the first line of the report that only sagittal and coronal views were taken. A third set of views called axial views are required to completely judge the position of the kneecap. These views are carried out in most MRI facilities.

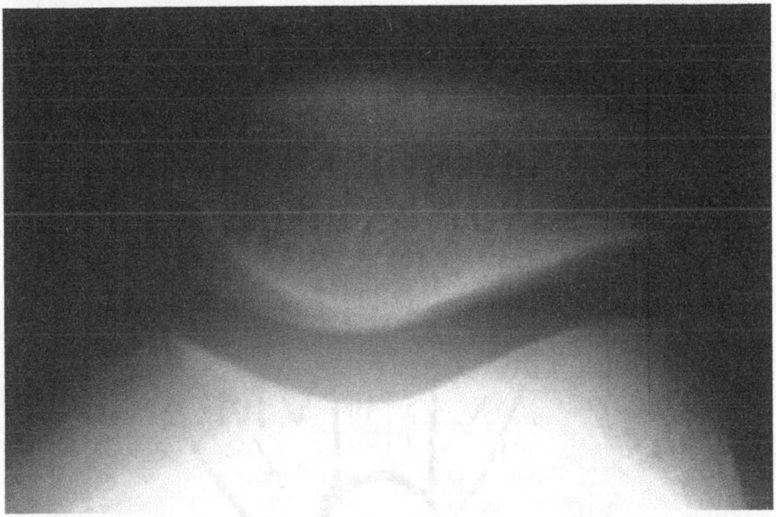

Figure 6-1. This is the "patellofemoral" compartment of the knee (as seen when you are looking down with your x-ray vision at your bent knee). "Patella" is the medical term for kneecap. Roundish when seen from the front, it is triangular in cross-section. It glides within the "trochlear groove" of the femur. The empty space is cartilage.

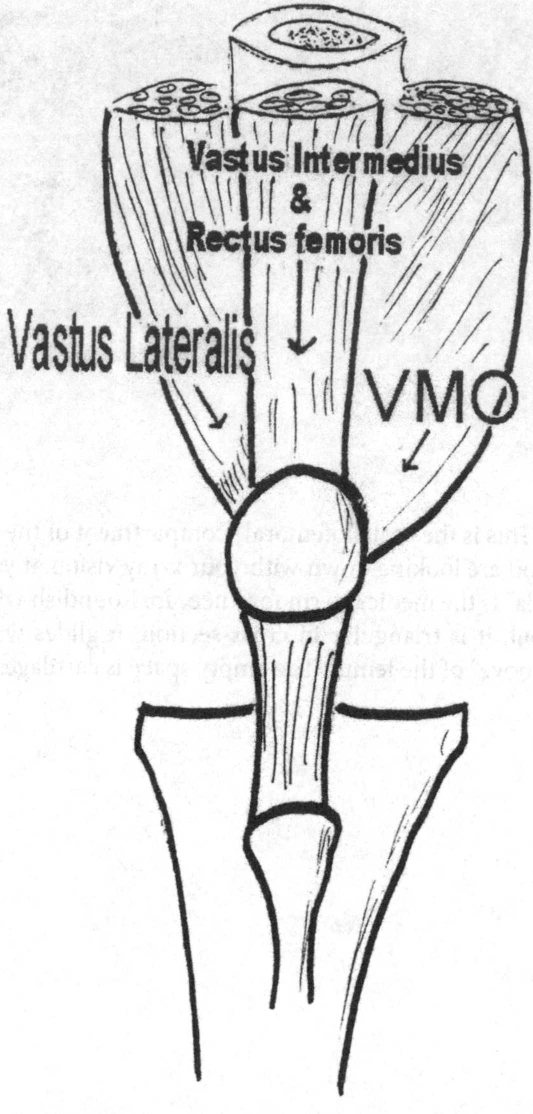

Figure 6-2. The quadriceps muscles. The vastus lateralis pulls the kneecap to the outside; the VMO (vastus medialis obliquus) pulls to the inside. The rectus femoris and vastus intermedius pull straight up.

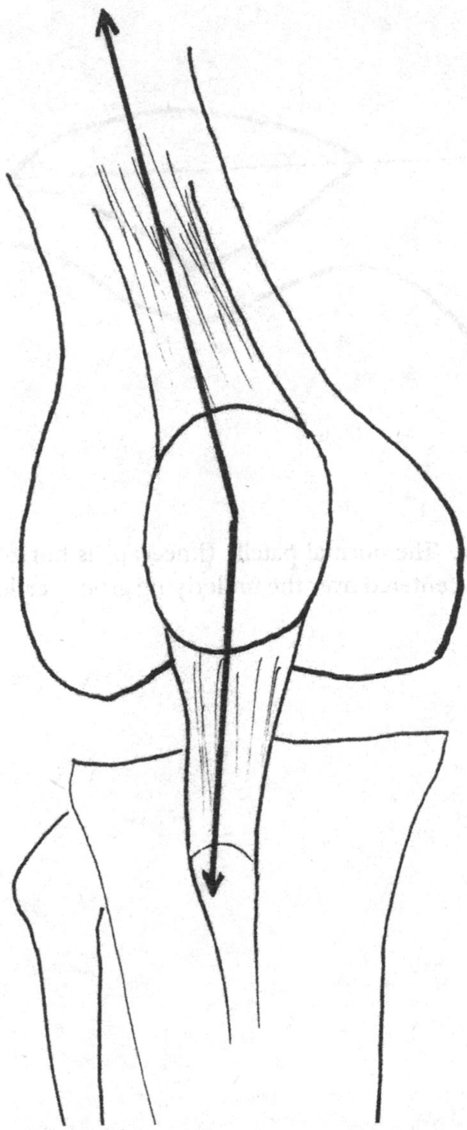

Figure 6-3. The quadriceps muscles and patellar tendon (a.k.a. ligament) form an angle—the Q angle. When the Q angle is excessive, contraction of the quads tends to pull the patella out of its groove.

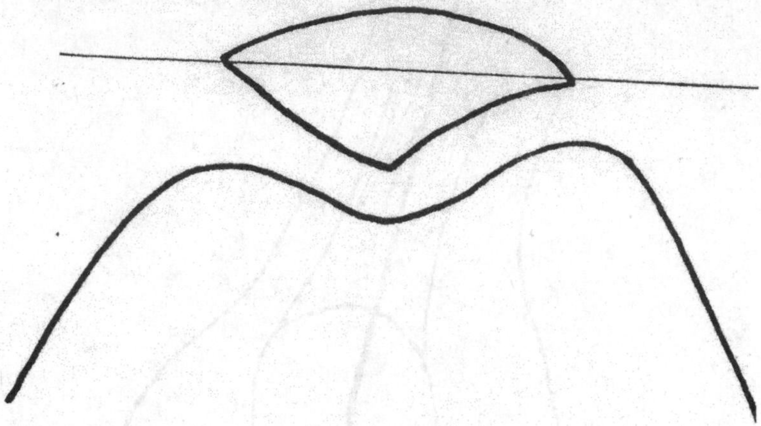

Figure 6-4a. The normal patella (kneecap) is horizontal—or nearly so. It is also centered over the underlying groove called the trochlea.

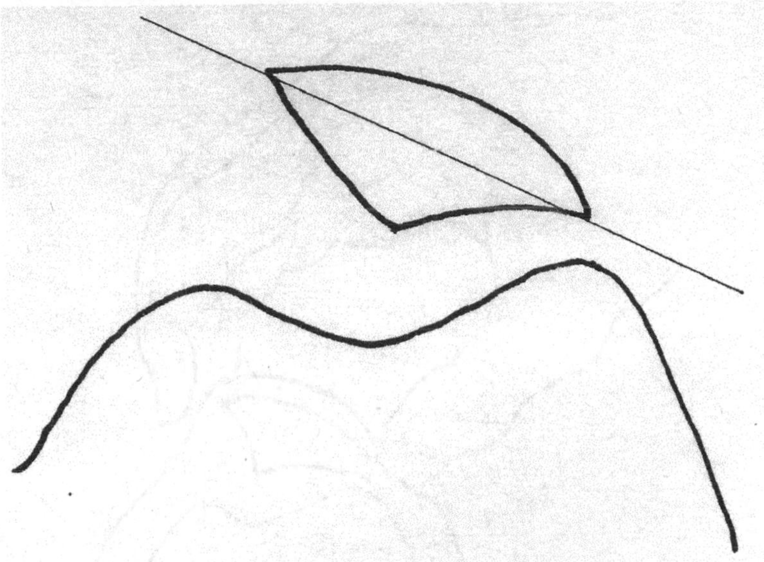

Figure 6-4b. A tilted patella is associated with a tight "lateral retinaculum" and can predispose to pain and/or instability.

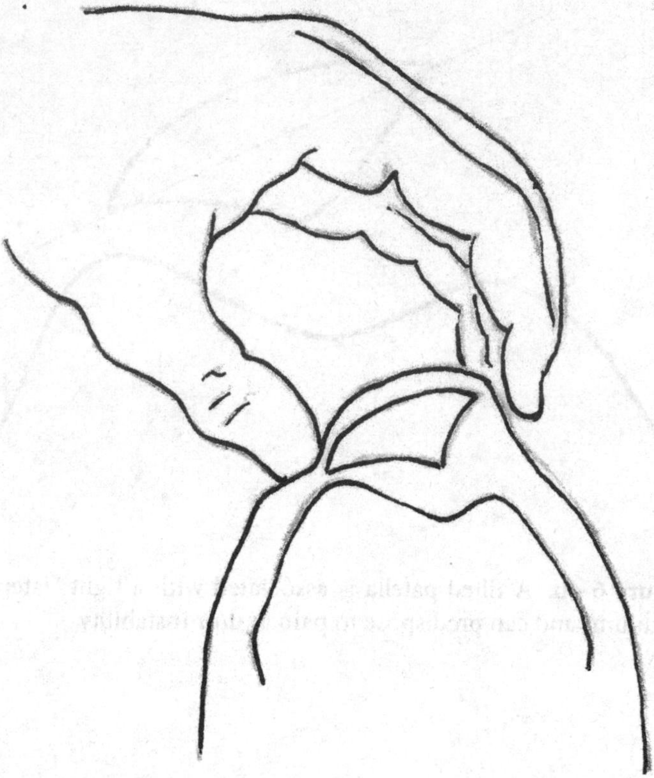

Figure 6-4c. It is easy for a knee doctor or physical therapist to check for tilting of the patella and tenderness of the lateral retinaculum.

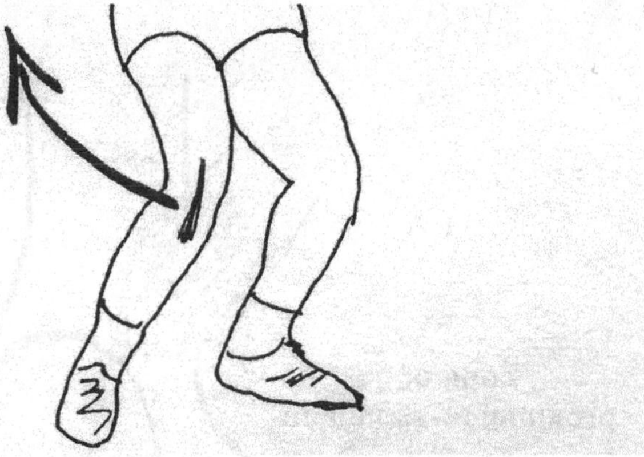

Figure 6-5. Twisting the upper body while keeping the feet planted on the ground can force the kneecap out of its groove. This can happen in athletes and recreational dancers—or can happen with a misstep.

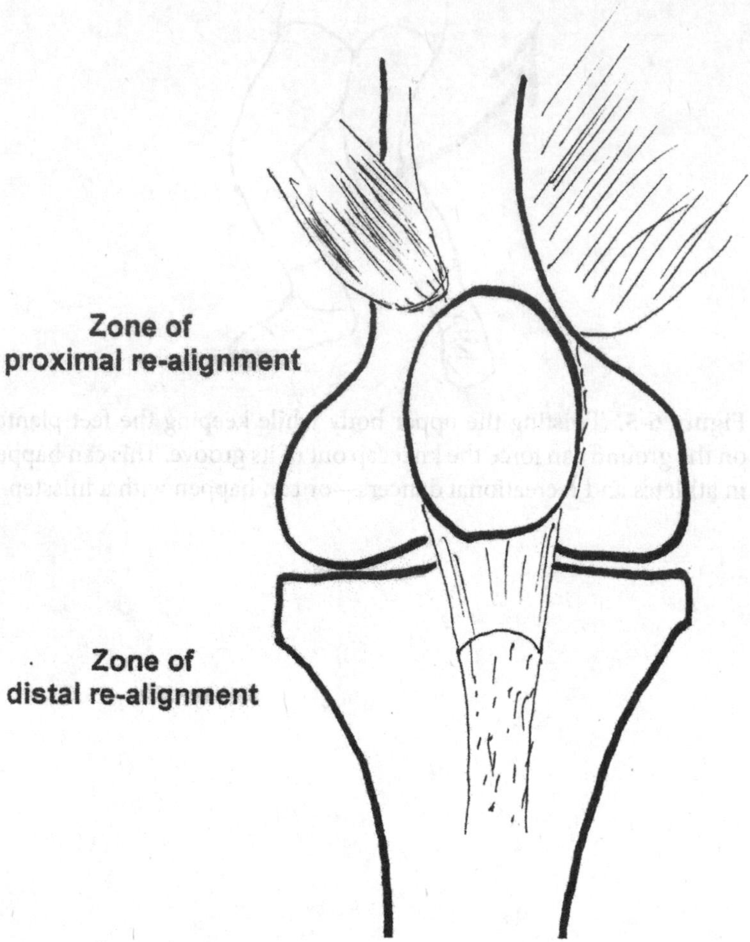

Figure 6-6. Operations that realign the kneecap are divided into proximal and distal procedures.

CHAPTER 7

The Hidden Causes of Knee Pain—Part 2

Summary Soundbite:

- A normal MRI doesn't mean there's nothing wrong with you.

A number of painful knee conditions will escape detection if the treating doctor relies solely on the MRI to make a diagnosis. In Chapter 6, we reviewed the large subject of pain pertaining to the kneecap. In this chapter, we will discuss equally painful and equally hidden sources of knee pain.

Tightness of the ITB

ITB stands for iliotibial band. This tough strap of tissue runs from the outer aspect of the upper leg, down the outside of the thigh, across the knee joint, and into the upper tibia (shinbone) (Figure 7-1). It fulfills a remarkable number of functions, one of which is to keep you from looking bow-legged every time you take a step. It is partly connected to your kneecap. The ITB is prone to tightness, and a number of painful conditions may ensue: the ITB can rub against the side of the femur (thighbone) giving rise to runner's knee (see below), it can contribute to pulling the kneecap off to the side, and it can alter the mechanics of the knee in painful fashion.

The diagnosis of a tight ITB is easy to make: the patient is placed on his/her side, the hips are extended (taken out of the flexed [bent] position), and the doctor notes whether or not the upper leg can be lowered to the examination table; this is called the Ober test. If the upper leg fails to come down to the table, the ITB is too tight.

Most patients with a painfully tight ITB can be treated with a stretching program supervised by a physical therapist (see Figure 11-6). But someone has to have made the diagnosis!

All too often, the doctor skips this time-consuming little test and goes right for the MRI; but a tight ITB does not show up on an MRI. What shows up instead is the ubiquitous reading of a torn meniscus, and yes, here we go again, a doctor may recommend surgery.

Tendinitis/Runner's Knee

There are tendons everywhere about the knee and they can become painfully irritated. The pain comes on with the bending and straightening of the knee, and if the condition is severe enough, the pain can even be present at rest. Usually the diagnosis is made by palpating the painful area. Again, this requires some attention on the part of the examining physician. Note once more that tendinitis of the knee does not routinely show up on an MRI. You will therefore be misdiagnosed by any practitioner who relies exclusively on the MRI.

Two of the most commonly irritated tendons are the iliotibial band (ITB) and the patellar tendon.

Runner's Knee. Runner's knee is the name given to an inflammation of the lower part of the ITB just as it crosses the upper part of the knee (see Figure 7-1). In the susceptible person, it comes from repeatedly bending the knee back and forth. It happens perhaps most commonly in runners, but just as tennis elbow isn't limited to tennis players, runner's knee can afflict cyclists, soccer players, lacrosse players, and just about any athlete who runs.

The pain is localized to the lower-most part of the outer thigh, right over the knobby part of the knee. Typically, the pain doesn't kick in until the runner has reached a certain mileage ("Doc, I'm fine until I reach 2.5 miles"), and it quiets down with rest. It also hurts when you press right over the outer aspect of the knee. If you suspect that this is what you are suffering from, try an ITB stretching program (see Figure 11-6), make sure you've warmed up before running, and for two weeks or so, consider taking an over-the-counter anti-inflammatory medication such as ibuprofen or naproxen prior to running. If your knee still hurts when you come home from running, applying a cold pack to the painful area can calm the pain. When running, temporarily cut back to mileage that doesn't hurt; or switch to swimming for a week or two if you can. Then gradually work up the mileage.

I haven't found braces to be particularly useful for runner's knee, but if a friend of yours has one, try it. It won't do you any harm. Avoid running along the side of the hill (it makes you run crooked), and make sure your shoes aren't worn down. In fact, think back to whether your pain started when you bought your latest running shoes. Every shoe turns your foot in or out in an ever so slightly different way, and sometimes that's enough to throw off your knee mechanics. So if the start of your pain coincided with your latest shoe purchase, try a model that resembles your old shoes. Are you flatfooted; are your arches high? Think about a consultation with a podiatrist for full-length shoe orthotics (devices you slip into a shoe).

<u>Patellar tendinitis.</u> The patellar tendon connects the kneecap (patella) to the tibia (shinbone). It can become irritated in athletes who repeatedly jump. The pain and tenderness are localized to the lower part of the kneecap or to the area just below. Treatment involves (yikes) holding off on that basketball playing until things quiet down. As with any tendinitis, adjunctive management includes anti-inflammatory medication and physical therapy for the application of ultrasound and related treatments. If the tendinitis is so severe that it interferes with everyday activities, you may

need a brace that doesn't let you bend the knee: a knee immobilizer. Indeed every time you bend the knee, you are tugging on the kneecap and on the tendon connecting the kneecap to the shinbone. By preventing this, you allow the tendinitis to quiet down.

In some people, a small area of tendon can spontaneously lose its blood supply. It feels the same as tendinitis, but it is technically referred to as tendin*osis*. This particular variation of tendinitis doesn't respond well to anti-inflammatory medication. (Inflammation isn't part of the picture.) Orthopedists occasionally treat tendinosis by surgically excising the involved area.

Just about every tendon is a candidate for tendinitis. The initial treatment is the same in all cases: avoidance of painful activities, a trial of anti-inflammatory medication (if you are allowed these), and physical therapy to gently stretch and soothe the painful area.

Fat pad inflammation

Behind your patellar tendon lies a large glob of fat that becomes apparent when you straighten the knee. It looks like two separate bumps, but it's just one, the middle of which has been pushed down by the tendon. It can become irritated.

The difficulty lies not with the treatment, but, as with so many other conditions in this chapter, with the diagnosis. A radiologist is not likely to make the diagnosis for you. It's up to your doctor to examine you. The initial treatment is the same as with all other soft tissue irritations: rest, anti-inflammatory medication, activity modification, physical therapy, injection . . .

What is a neuroma?

Quite a simple condition, actually. There are thousands of small nerves around the knee that supply sensation to the skin: these are the nerves that let you know when something is touching your knee. Some of these nerves are visible to the naked eye, others not. By and large they are branches of the saphenous nerve that runs along the inner thigh. When these nerves are bruised, they send pain signals to the brain. Under the microscope you can sometimes see swelling or scarring of the nerves. However, bruised nerves and neuromas are by and large not revealed on an MRI. The diagnosis is easy to make on a physical examination: if the skin hurts when it is lightly squeezed, when a thumbnail is gently run along it, or when it is gently tapped, you might have a neuroma. Injecting a little local anesthetic under the skin confirms the diagnosis. The treatment involves physical therapy for desensitization or injecting a combination of an anesthetic and a specialized steroid medication. Two or three injections might be required, and if this does not work, the affected tissue under the skin of the affected area might need to be surgically removed. The result is an area of numbness—usually a welcome trade for the person who has gone so far as to require surgery. (Note that these special steroid injections can cause localized whitening of the skin.)

Considering how easy it is to diagnose a neuroma, I am surprised at how often the diagnosis is missed.

Without there being an actual, visible neuroma, the saphenous nerve can nevertheless be painfully irritated, in which case the technical term would be neuritis.

Falling onto one's knee or striking one's knee against the dashboard of a car is a common mechanism for developing a neuroma/neuritis.

Core Insufficiency

Control of the legs starts with the muscles around the abdomen and buttocks. When these muscles are weak and/or abnormally tight, knee pain can ensue. Modern physical therapy regimens are geared toward evaluation and treatment of the core structures.

Reflex Sympathetic Dystrophy (RSD) / (CRPS Complex Regional Pain Syndrome (CRPS)

This is a disorder of the nervous system that can cause severe pain. Imagine someone placing pepper under your nose. You would sneeze. With the pepper removed, the sneezing would stop. Imagine now sneezing on indefinitely even with the pepper removed. RSD is similar in that pain persists long after the inciting event has gone.

RSD is an incompletely appreciated condition. The first English-language documentation of the condition dates back to the American Civil War. It goes by a number of names including causalgia, shoulder-hand syndrome (when it occurs in the arm), Sudeck's atrophy, sympathetically maintained pain, and complex regional pain syndrome (CRPS). Specialists in this area will tell you that there are subtle differences between these conditions, but by and large, they all consist of persistent, painful misfiring of pain fibers. It is unknown at this point why a small number of people develop this "reflex," but we know that just about anything can trigger the condition: a twist, a sprain, a surgical procedure of any kind, neurological disorders, cancer, and so forth. In its full blown, classic incarnation, RSD presents with exquisite burning and unrelenting pain to even the lightest touch. Pants and bed sheets are intolerable. The skin is initially hot and then eventually very cool. It can be reddish, purplish, or mottled. The affected joint is stiff, and the affected limb can become atrophic (skinny) and dysfunctional (i.e., dystrophic).

RSD is a condition of variable expression as not every patient presents with the classic picture. In its most elemental form, RSD can simply consist of undue pain.

The best test for RSD is a sympathetic block. This is an injection administered just to side of the spine (usually by an anesthesiologist), and it is designed to block the sympathetic nerves to the affected area. These nerves are part of the "autonomic" nervous system that controls body functions that are not under voluntary control (e.g., breathing, digesting). When these nerves are blocked with Novocain® or an equivalent numbing medication, the patient with RSD suddenly feels warmth in the extremity and a relief of pain. Because the cause of sympathetic misfiring is not known, multiple treatments exist, and each targets a slightly different site along the neurological pathway. These treatments include pills, injections, and physical therapy. The key to treatment, regardless of the strategy chosen, is to institute it early, as RSD addressed early on tends to respond better and more quickly. Unfortunately, because RSD often presents in subtle forms, it can escape detection for long periods of time.

Referred Pain

The body is funny in that pain in one part of the body can actually be caused by a problem far removed. Shoulder pain, for example, can come from a sick gallbladder or a pinched nerve in the neck. Likewise, pain around the knee can come from the hip, pelvis, or back. Note: no *knee* MRI will detect a hip or back problem.

Children are particularly prone to having hip problems manifesting only as knee pain, but it can happen at any age. On average, I see two patients a year in need of hip replacement surgery whose only symptoms are about the knee. More commonly, a pinched nerve in the lower back will cause radiating pain in the knee. This may not be associated with any back pain. When the clinical and radiographic examination of the knee is perfectly normal—or not abnormal enough to account for the severity of knee symptoms—the doctor will turn his or her attention to other causes of knee pain including the referred pain just described. Things become more difficult when there *are* enough findings about the knee to account for the knee pain. The doctor treats those findings (sometimes for quite a long time), and then, to everyone's dismay, the original symptoms persist. They do so because the knee findings were only part of the problem to begin with. Let me quickly point out that when this happens, it doesn't automatically mean that the doctor has been ignorant or negligent. However, faced with someone with persistent, unexplained knee pain, the surgeon at some point has to start looking elsewhere.

The following entities are not likely to be missed, but it may take a while for the diagnosis to become clear. This is especially true if the conditions do not manifest themselves in a classic manner.

Osgood-Schlatter's

Often pronounced "osgoodschlitis" by the public, this condition was described by two separate doctors a continent apart (you guessed it: Osgood and Schlatter). It consists of a painful swelling at the upper shin, and as painful as it is, it is not serious. It occurs most often in young teenagers (a week before they're to leave for summer camp, of course) and it tends to improve on its own over time. The problem is that neither the child nor the parents are usually in the mood to simply wait it out. It is therefore worth trying a number of nonoperative measures such as activity modification, anti-inflammatory medication, physical therapy, and knee braces. None of these approaches comes close to being 100 percent effective; Osgood-Schlatter's leads to many second opinions.

In my experience, some teenagers suffering from Osgood-Schlatter's also have a high-riding kneecap (patella alta), and this aspect of the condition may go undetected. When there is such an associated disorder, it is worth reviewing it with the family. It would be important for the parents to know, for example, that their child may have knee problems in the future. They may perhaps want to steer the child away from certain athletic activities. This is part of an "informed consumer" discussion. At the very least, the family will believe their child when he or she complains of pain.

Bursitis

A bursa is a structure commonly found around joints—especially the large joints such as the knee, hip, and shoulder. In its normal state, it is akin to a small oily balloon, and it helps to provide smooth, painless motion about joints. When inflamed, a bursa turns into a water balloon. It swells and becomes painful. The condition is called "bursitis." Around the knee, the bursa most likely to become inflamed is the one that lies over the kneecap. The diagnosis is easy to make because there is such obvious swelling directly over the front of the knee. The bursa can become inflamed as a result of direct trauma, for example landing directly onto the knee;

the bursa fills with blood. The bursa can also become inflamed as a result of repeated rubbing, as when working on one's knees. Here the fluid is likely to be yellow and not bloody.

The treatment depends on how much swelling is present and how much pain the patient is in. At one extreme, the condition can be observed, and at the other, a needle is placed into the distended bursa and the fluid is aspirated (drawn out). Occasionally, the fluid continues to re-accumulate, and surgery is required to remove part of the bursa and allow the tissues to scar down.

Rheumatism

This commonly used term doesn't actually exist in the world of medicine. There are, however, a host of rheumatological conditions within the world of rheumatology. These include a large number of nontraumatic afflictions of joints and muscles such as rheumatoid arthritis, psoriatic arthritis, lupus, Reiter's syndrome, and gout—to name but a few. These are all disorders affecting the entire body. Not every part of the body need be symptomatic though, and the pain can start in just one area, for example, the knee. When one of these conditions is present, one or more blood tests will be abnormal. For instance, when a person suffers from gout, the uric acid level is elevated, and in rheumatoid arthritis, the rheumatoid factor and sedimentation rate are elevated. Early on, nevertheless, all tests can be normal. An increasing number of rheumatological diseases are associated with genetic markers, and a rheumatologist is the expert to discuss these topics with. Classically, rheumatological conditions (also known as "inflammatory" conditions) present with swelling, heat and redness about the knee, and occasionally a generalized fever—but not necessarily. Sometimes, the knee simply hurts.

Lyme Disease (and other tick-borne conditions such as Ehrlichiosis and Babesia)

Lyme disease features a typical rash, but the rash is fleeting. Thereafter, Lyme can manifest itself in a myriad of ways—knee pain being one. Tuberculosis used to be called "The Great Impersonator" owing to its multiple presentations; in the western world, Lyme disease is the new "Great Impersonator." It is relatively rare compared to the conditions listed above and will not be at the top of anybody's list; it may not make it at all onto an orthopedist's list.

When testing for rheumatism, it's now common to test for Lyme and related conditions.

Bone "Strokes" (Osteochondritis Dissecans Avascular Necrosis)

Some of the more mysterious conditions about the knee involve a loss of blood flow to a part of the bone (usually the femur [thighbone]). In that sense, I liken them to a stroke. In adolescents and young adults, the condition goes by the name of osteochondritis dissecans (abbreviated OCD), and in adults it is called osteonecrosis or avascular necrosis (a.k.a. aseptic necrosis, AVN) (see Figure 7-2). AVN usually occurs in adults who are between fifty-five and seventy-five. Women are more at risk.

OCD is treated nonoperatively in young teenagers, but usually requires surgery in older teenagers and adults. The younger the patient, the better the prognosis. In AVN a segment of bone does literally die. The segment can be small and the patient can recover quite well, or it can be large and eventually require major surgery. Most significantly, from a diagnostic point of view, the pain can come out of the blue. The person develops sudden, intense knee pain for no apparent reason. Although I have previously stated that MRIs are vastly over prescribed, the onset of sudden knee pain in someone over the age of fifty-five is a good indication for an MRI if x-rays are unremarkable.

Pigmented Villonodular Synovitis (PVNS)/ Osteochondromatosis

The knee is lined with a glistening layer of tissue, in the same way that all the walls of a room might be covered with carpeting.

This lining is called synovium. In normal conditions, it secretes a small amount of fluid (synovial fluid) which, among other things, provides lubrication for the joint. Tumors can grow from this synovial tissue, and secrete abnormal, bloody fluid (as in pigmented villonodular synovitis, or PVNS) and even bits of tissue resembling grains of rice (osteochondromatosis). These conditions are not visible on an x-ray. The diagnosis is made on an MRI or is revealed at the time of an arthroscopy. These are not cancerous conditions: they do not spread to other parts of the body. They can involve just a small part of the knee or a major portion of it. They can be relatively indolent or can be aggressive, in which case they grow quickly and destroy the tissues in their immediate vicinity. They are usually well treated by an arthroscopy (see Chapter 3), but the more aggressive tumors recur.

Infection

Infections can occur anywhere in the body, including the knee. The typical infection causes pain, swelling, redness, and a fever. This can also be the presentation of gout and other rheumatisms and is therefore a potential source of confusion. Infections about the knee are treated with antibiotics. The knee may also be aspirated (fluid removed with a needle) or washed out in the operating room by means of an arthroscopy. A rare cause of infection in the knee is tuberculosis, which in the United States, is likely to be unrecognized for a long time.

Tumors

Tumors exist about the knee as they can anywhere else in the body. They are divided into those that are malignant (cancerous) and those that are benign. Benign tumors cause damage in the area where they grow, but by and large, do not spread to other parts of the body. The list of potential tumors about the knee is remarkably long. Fortunately, if your doctor suspects a tumor, there are a number of tests available today that will provide a rapid diagnosis.

Summary:

Mysterious knee pain often simply requires a thorough examination of your knee. An MRI is a poor substitute for a hasty examination.

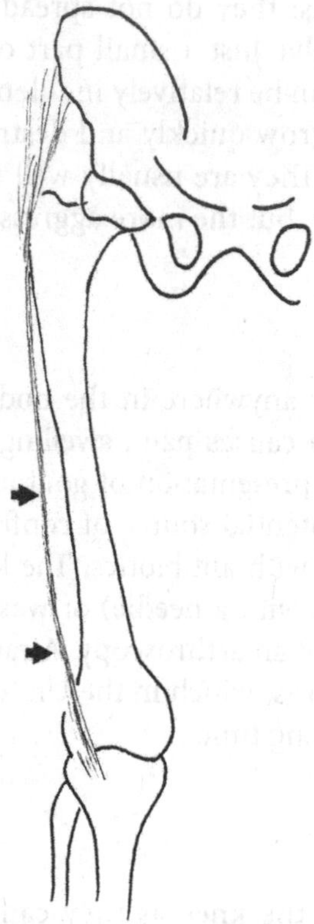

Figure 7-1. The arrows point to the ITB (iliotibial band) that goes from the ilium (pelvis) down to the upper tibia. It can rub against the lower (or upper) femur with repetitive knee bending and straightening. At the knee this can cause the iliiotibial friction syndrome, sometimes called "runner's knee."

CHAPTER 8

Does Anyone Here Know How to Take an X-Ray?

Summary Soundbite:

- Knee x-rays have become a lost art. Expect them to make a comeback.

Contrary to what you might have been led to believe, a vast amount of information can be obtained from x-rays—provided that the appropriate views are obtained and provided that the quality of the pictures is reasonable.

Nevertheless, by and large, patients undergo suboptimal x-rays and are then immediately sent for an MRI. It is true that, on occasion, an MRI provides critical nuggets of information that could never have been detected on x-rays. More commonly though, the MRI provides information that can be obtained from a physical examination and plain x-rays. You might also be surprised to find that plain x-rays can occasionally provide information *not* found on an MRI. Finally, it is not uncommon, in the setting of knee pain, for the MRI to be frankly misleading (see Chapter 2).

Unless you are being x-rayed in an orthopedist's office, chances are that the x-rays obtained will be of the so-called AP and lateral type. AP stands for anteroposterior. This means that the x-ray beam is going from front to back. A lateral is a side view. These two x-rays represent a mug shot of your knee. They are quickly performed and they are inexpensive. They are adequate for detecting major fractures and moderate to severe arthritis. For this reason, these are the views obtained in an emergency room. For many patients, though, these x-rays are inadequate.

Arthritis by definition is a wearing down of the cartilage lining the ends of bones. When this wearing down occurs over a significant portion of the knee, the bones come close to touching each other on an x-ray, and this can be seen on the routine AP x-ray described above. However, because the person is lying down, this narrowing of the joint may be missed and better appreciated in a standing position. When joint space narrowing is identified, the diagnosis of arthritis is made, and an MRI becomes superfluous (see below).

In more subtle cases, the location of the arthritis within the knee dictates not just that the person be standing but that the knees be bent during the taking of the x-ray. This has been called the Rosenberg view (or standing flexion view or schuss view, a crude reference to the position of a schussing skier) (Figures 8-1 and 8-2). Anyone middle-aged or older should undergo this view. Again, if narrowing of the space between the bones is detected, the diagnosis is made and an MRI is completely unnecessary. Compared to the cost of an MRI, a Rosenberg view is practically free. (Note: the setup for this view is best performed by an x-ray technician who frequently takes knee x-rays.)

Arthritis is not the only condition that can be diagnosed on an x-ray. More unusual conditions such as osteochondritis dissecans (OCD) and avascular necrosis (see Chapter 7) can also be detected. These conditions occasionally require a so-called tunnel view: with the patient lying on the x-ray table, an x-ray is taken with the knee bent about 45 degrees. If you will, this is a Rosenberg view taken with the patient lying down. (The tunnel view is easier for the technician than the Rosenberg view.) Bone spurs will occasionally lie in parts of the knee only visible on a tunnel view.

The front of the knee is one of the most common areas of knee pain, and poor positioning of the kneecap can be a factor (see Chapter 6). When the medical history and the examination point to this, an x-ray can help identify the diagnosis. Again, inexpensive but appropriate views need to be obtained. These views include a true lateral (Figure 8-3) and a Merchant view (Figure 8-4) (see Chapter 6).

A true lateral (side view)—as opposed to the garden-variety type rapidly obtained in an Emergency Room—is taken perpendicular to the end of the thighbone, and requires a little practice and perseverance on the part of the x-ray technician. This is the best view for assessing from top to bottom the groove your kneecap glides in (the trochlea) (see Chapter 6).

The Merchant view involves draping the knees over a simple device that is placed at the end of the x-ray table. (It costs just half an MRI.) The device keeps the knees bent a specific number of degrees, most commonly 30 or 45 degrees (see Figure 8-4). The less bent the better, for kneecap malalignment is best detected with the knee just slightly bent. Without this view, it is impossible to make a preliminary assessment of the kneecap's left-right position or tilting, and difficult to judge the presence of arthritis. If the medical history, the physical examination, and the x-ray strongly point to the kneecap, no MRI is necessary at this point, and the patient can safely be treated for the kneecap issue. Such problems usually improve with simple, nonoperative programs (see Chapter 6).

What is wrong with simply getting an MRI?

It is expensive—and it doesn't always give you all the requisite information—and it can be misleading—and it can lead to unnecessary surgery. Add up the cost of all the unnecessary MRIs in the US and you get a hefty figure. This cost affects your premiums and it affects the insurance companies' ability to pay for truly useful tests and treatments.

Appropriate x-rays often suffice.

The MRI can miss conditions that an x-ray will detect. Indeed, the MRI is performed with the patient lying down, muscles relaxed. This is not the position in which a knee usually hurts! Arthritis can be missed on a low-quality MRI even when detected on the standing AP or Rosenberg view.

Another condition often missed on an MRI is chondrocalcinosis. This mouthful of a condition simply translates to "cartilage calcium," that is, calcium in the cartilage. As important as it is to have calcium in bones, it does not belong in cartilage! When present in cartilage, microscopic knife-like calcium crystals are released into the knee. This can cause painful swelling. Although the abnormal calcium is clearly visible on x-rays, it often is not apparent on an MRI.

As we've seen now many times throughout this book, the MRI can be terribly misleading. Some radiology centers routinely read a torn meniscus on every MRI. This can be done out of ignorance or malice (where the intent is to get more business from orthopedists and personal injury attorneys). In any case, such a finding often focuses the attention of the patient onto an irrelevant issue. An MRI in a patient whose knee is known to be arthritic, for example, adds little if any useful information, and usually it will not (should not) affect treatment. (As noted on page 26, even the discovery of a torn meniscus should not affect the treatment.) The patient will be treated (should be treated) nonoperatively at first, regardless of what the MRI shows and will be treated surgically if the nonoperative treatment fails. This will be true regardless of the MRI findings.

Is there ever a good reason for obtaining an MRI?

Of course. The MRI is an extraordinary test. When the doctor is truly stumped, an MRI can reveal subtle and rare conditions such as tumors. If there has been a major injury to the knee and surgery is being contemplated, the MRI can help assess the status of "soft tissues" such as the cruciate ligaments. If a patient suffers from kneecap malalignment and even the Merchant view and true lateral are normal, an MRI can sometimes detect this malalignment. If a patient is found to have OCD (see Chapter 7), the MRI can be of use in planning surgery. If an older patient has the early stages of osteonecrosis (a bone stroke—see Chapter 7), this might only be detected on an MRI.

If surgery is about to be performed for, say, a truly torn cartilage, an MRI can be obtained to insure that there is no other problem in the knee. This practice of obtaining an MRI "just to make sure there is nothing else going on" is an expensive one considering how rare it is to find something on the MRI that will change the surgeon's mind. Still, in the United States it is an acceptable use of the MRI. (In other countries it is not acceptable. This means that we are either particularly prudent or particularly spendthrift.)

Take Home Message: In a large number of patients with knee pain, quality x-rays obviate the need for MRI imaging.

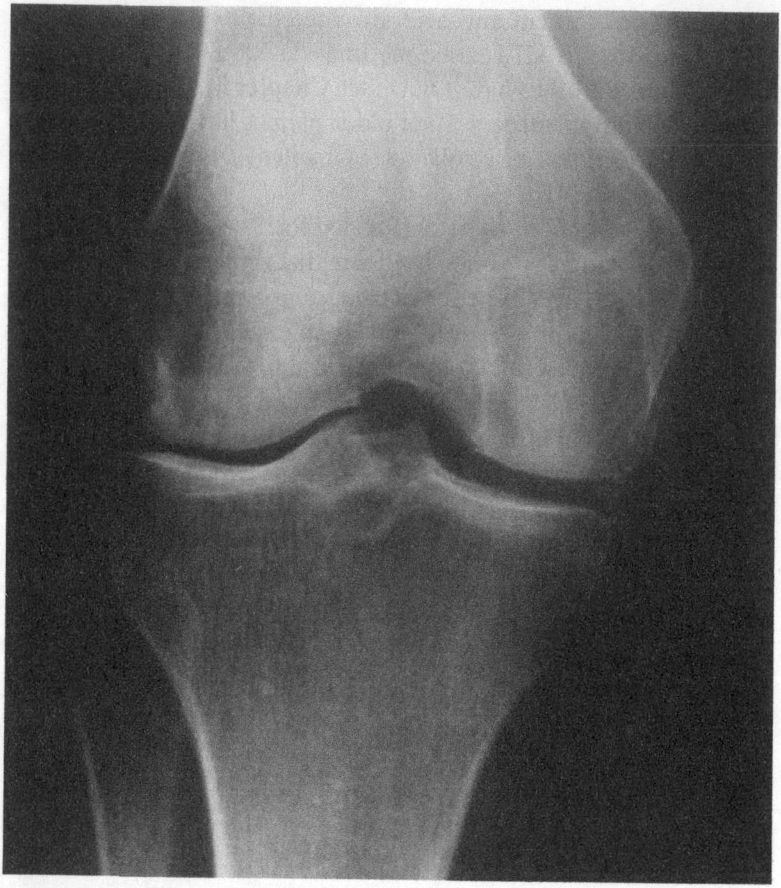

Figure 8-1. This x-ray has been taken with the patient standing. It is an improvement relative to a supine (lying down) x-ray. Note the narrowing of the lateral (outside) compartment (on the left here). This indicates wear of the articular cartilage. A doctor may suggest an MRI to check for a torn meniscus. This would not be necessary.

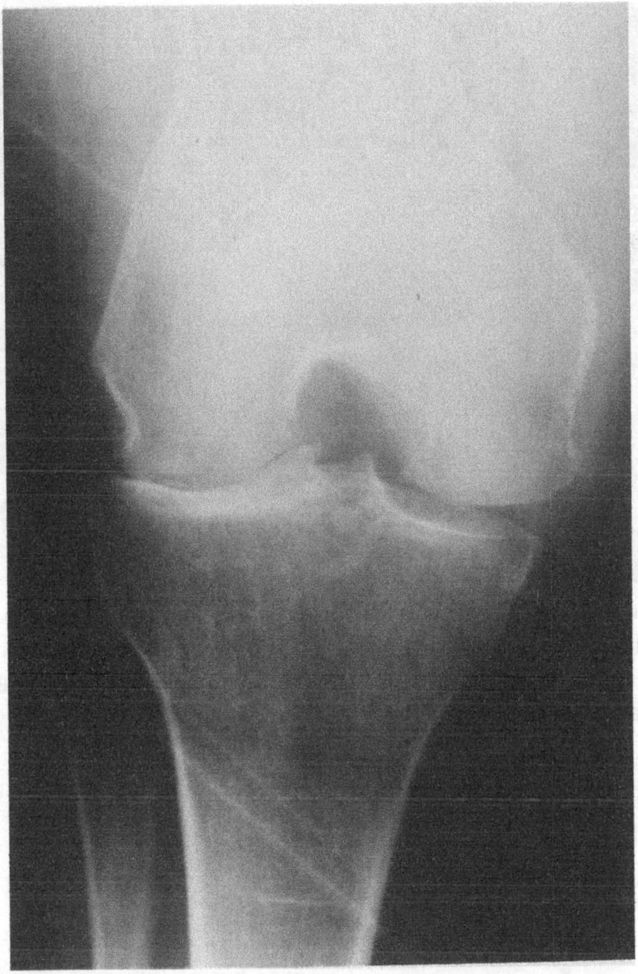

Figure 8-2. Even better, the standing x-ray has now been taken with the knees bent. Note the obliteration of the joint space. There IS no articular cartilage left. The meniscus caught between the two surfaces is indeed most likely frayed and torn, but a) no MRI is needed to make that call and b) a tear in this setting is irrelevant (see text). There is no need for an MRI.

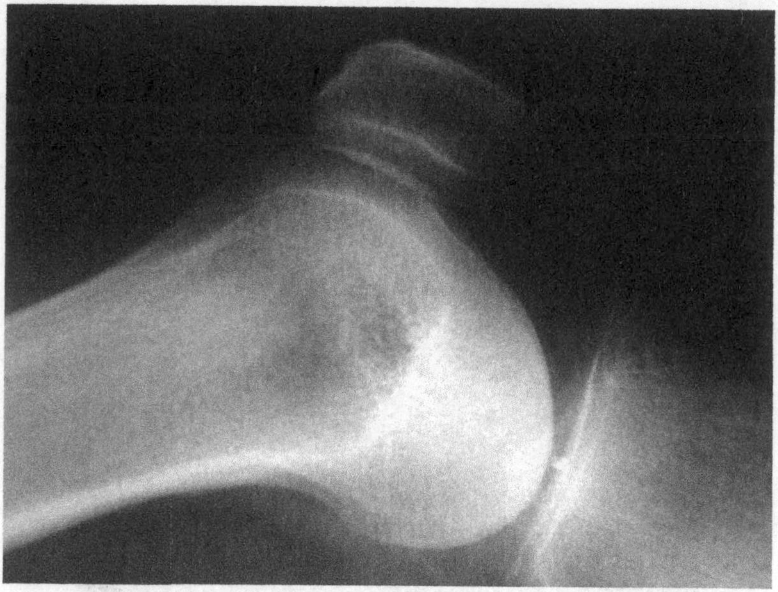

Figure 8-3. A TRUE lateral of the knee. The condyles (knobs) at the end of the thighbone overlap nearly perfectly giving the appearance of a "one condyle" knee. With a such a view, your doctor can make critical evaluations of the trochlear groove (see Chapter 6).

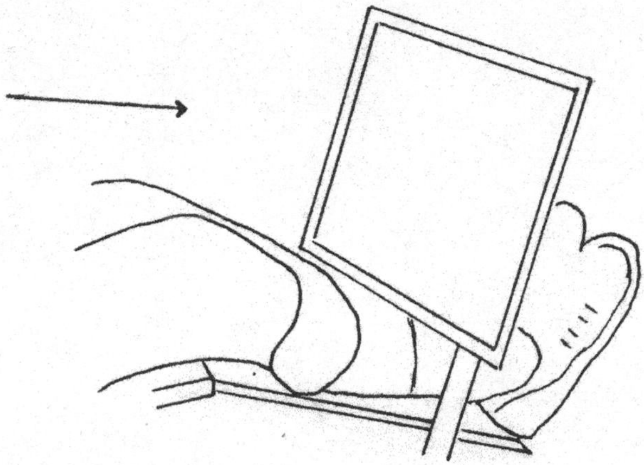

Figure 8-4. The Merchant view is used to see whether the kneecap is out of alignment and/or arthritic. Ideally, the knee is bent no more than 30 degrees. The cost of the equipment needed is half the cost of a single MRI.

CHAPTER 9
The Placebo: A Misunderstood Treatment

"The line between treatment and placebo is blurrier than ever."
—Neurologist M. Okun in "Mind Over Matter,"
National Geographic, December 2016.

The wonderful placebo effect

A placebo is the strangest treatment of them all. The moment a patient discovers its method of action, it stops working. A placebo is a treatment recognized as having no clear medical benefit—other than the patient's satisfaction at having received a concrete form of attention.

The word placebo comes from the Latin, meaning "I please you." The implication is that the treatment does nothing but satisfy the patient's need for medical attention. Remarkably, sometimes that's all it takes to make the problem go away! Therefore, it really *is* a treatment. Placebo is sometimes used synonymously with "doesn't work, it's just there to fool you," and that is simply not correct. Well, not completely correct. It does indeed fool you, but it *can* be effective.

Here's the a placebo mechanism: the mere fact that a person believes in a treatment somehow makes it effective. You gotta believe. "Mind over matter" you might say. Naturally, the more a person believes, the better the placebo effect.

At jury duty a while back, the officer who was reviewing policies and procedures to the huddled masses in front of him made the following announcement: "The water fountain has a foot pedal and a button. Ignore the pedal. It's just a placebo. It doesn't work." Everybody laughed, but that pedal was no placebo. Had the pedal truly been a placebo, one-third of prospective jurors would have found that pushing that pedal had quenched their thirst!

Fully one-third of people will get pain relief from any pill. There are many ways to look at this: it's wonderful that an inexpensive tablet can help so many patients. On the other hand, look at the amount of money spent on medications that are no more effective than a placebo.

And we haven't talked about risks yet.

"My friend Mary takes Pain-Go-Away for her knee and she thinks it's terrific. Stopped her pain like that!" So starts many a conversation. Patients not uncommonly come to the office hoping that I will prescribe the same medication their friend has. It's not necessarily unreasonable. The fact that Mary feels great with Pain-Go-Away only predisposes my patient that much more toward getting a placebo benefit. On the other hand, if there are medications that are more effective than Pain-Go-Away, it's unreasonable not to take the better medication.

One of the remarkable findings is that aggressive, invasive treatments such as surgery also have a placebo effect. This is especially true of certain operations designed to alleviate pain, and it applies particularly to the knee. In a very limited study (not involving any of my patients) patients with knee pain underwent a sham arthroscopy. (For this procedure, small holes [portals] are made at the front of the knee. Pencil-like instruments are placed into the knee through the portals, and these instruments are used to address whatever perceived problems exist in the knee.) For the purposes of this study, surgeons only made the two little portals. No instruments were inserted into the knee. I think anyone would agree that making two holes in the knee has no medicinal effect unless we're back to releasing evil humors. Yet, behold: some of the subjects reported feeling better! It is hard to know what aspect of the treatment provided the placebo effect. Being wheeled into the operating room? The intravenous in the arm? The anesthesia? The surgical pain from the two incisions? The confidence in the surgeon? The relief of really being taken seriously? Or maybe it's the whole package. As surprising as this finding might be, it really isn't so astonishing if you consider again how a placebo works: the subject needs to be impressed and to believe. The bigger the treatment, the more expensive the pill, the more well-known the doctor, the more impressionable the patient, the greater becomes the placebo effect. What bigger treatment is there than surgery?

Great Expectations

Once upon a time doctors knew nothing, yet they sounded as though they knew everything. There was a great deal of gentle deception. Not only was this socially acceptable, it was expected. Everybody suspected the doctors' very limited knowledge. It wasn't so long ago that doctors didn't know the difference between veins and arteries. In the days of Shakespeare, doctors had no clue as to why blood could be either dark red or bright red. The term "blood pressure" did not exist. As recently as 1860, Oliver Wendell Holmes is reported to have noted that if all medications "could be sunk to the bottom of the sea, it would be all the better for mankind—and all the worse for the fishes."[13] Nevertheless, the know-it-all attitude of doctors was critical to the placebo effect—the only effect that could be expected. Nowadays, doctors still don't come close to knowing everything, but they really do have a great deal of scientific, evidence-based medical information. Because of this new knowledge patients expect a cure every time. In the absence of mystery, patients want to be part of the decision making process. They want to be informed of choices and options. Whereas failure used to be the norm, success is now so common

---

[13] Talbot, M, "The Placebo Prescription," *New York Times Magazine*, January 9, 2000.

that failure has become unacceptable. Hence the lawsuits and the "I had no idea things could turn out so bad" frame of mind.

This brings up a tricky issue: informed consent. Patients in the United States want to be fully informed. And I agree with this completely. I certainly want to be fully informed before I agree to a procedure, medication, or treatment of any kind for that matter. Having said that, by the time a surgeon finishes talking about all the risks and all the potential complications, he's pretty much ruined any placebo effect he might have been counting on. In fact, now you've got a scared patient. Your patient is at risk for the reverse placebo effect! The subject is so frightened by the thought of a complication that recovery is compromised. If the placebo effect exists for the better, you have to believe that it can occur for the worse.

Given all this, how then does the surgeon explain a procedure to a patient? The surgeon is supposed to inform the patient of reasonable risks but it is up to the surgeon to decide what constitutes reasonable. There is no official catalogue of reasonable risks. I think you have to inform patients of any factor that could lead them to change their mind—but that can vary from patient to patient. Moreover, it's not just *what* the surgeon tells you it's *how* he tells you. He can rapidly go through the risks in a dismissive tone of voice or he can spell each one out in exquisite detail. In the former case, the surgeon is leading the patient down a falsely rosy path and in the latter he is sabotaging his own practice. Who wants to be operated on by a surgeon who spends so much time talking about complications? He must have a lot of complications to be dwelling on them so much. I've seen people leave their surgeon "because he's such a downer." But if there isn't enough preoperative explaining (or perceived explaining), a patient can say she wasn't adequately informed. Obviously, there is a happy medium, but you can see how tricky a balancing act it is. There is a fine line between being reassuring and being dismissive. The better doctors know how to walk that line.

Making things more complicated is the fact that some patients don't want to hear about complications. They know they will probably benefit from the planned procedure and don't want to hear anything negative. To an extent, this is understandable. This attitude keeps patients in a positive frame of mind. They recognize that they are impressionable and subconsciously don't want to be subject to the reverse placebo effect. Unfortunately, in today's legal climate it is impossible not to discuss potential complications.

Do you know why hospitals pay large sums of money to have one of their doctors anointed team doctor for a professional team? Placebo. Patients want to be treated by the doctor who treats their favorite athletes. That doctor has to be good, right? The patient now has just one degree of separation from their athletic hero! Their chest swells with pride at the mere thought of this association. They're psyched! Their knee has to get better. And the fact is, it often does. Then, they refer their friends.

The down side

So why do placebos get such a bad rap? Money, risks, and diversion.

Diversion. Effective treatments exist for many conditions. For example, if you've just had an outpatient knee operation, we know that certain medications will control the pain. If instead, someone offers you a placebo that by definition may or may not work, they are diverting you away from a sure thing.

This may not be serious when we are only dealing with pain. After all, you can always switch back to a proven pain medication. But it is certainly serious if you are treating an infection, a heart attack, cancer, or any other condition where time is critical. Serious harm can befall you if you waste precious time on a placebo. (This seems to have been an issue with Steve Jobs.)

Risks. It's one thing if a placebo is harmless, it's quite another if there are significant risks associated with its use. The Hippocratic oath taken by every medical student states, "And first do no harm." A little starch pill won't do you any harm nor will water with a small amount of FDA-approved coloring in it. But a pill that can affect your kidney or a treatment associated with surgical complications, these are quite another story. ALL medications have potential side effects, as of course does surgery. It's one thing to take a chance on a treatment that has a very good chance of working, it's another to take that same chance on a treatment with a much lower success rate.

Money. Somebody's paying for your treatment. It may even be you. In fact, it's definitely you. It's just a question of whether you are paying directly or via premiums to an insurance company or via taxes. No one minds paying for safe and effective treatments. Placebos, though, aren't predictable in their effectiveness. No insurance (including the government) wants to shell out money for those kinds of odds. Too bad in a way, because an expensive medication is going to have a better placebo effect than an inexpensive one! Think about it: What makes you feel better about your visit to the doctor? A prescription for "Naproxen 250 mg bid sig#30" on the doctor's formal prescription pad or a simple recommendation to take over-the-counter Aleve® twice a day? Yet the two are essentially the same.

Reality

The FDA does not give its seal of approval to pain medications that are recognized to be placebos. Why not? Easy: If you tell people that you are selling a placebo, the placebo effect will be lost! People have to believe it's real medication. And if you don't tell people it's a placebo, then you're guilty of deception. The government is not into that—at least not at this level.

Manufacturers of nutritional supplements don't have those qualms. A nutritional supplement is often a product found in nature. It hasn't been created by mankind. It is something you might ingest in common food products. These nutritional supplements generally fall outside the purview of the FDA. Manufacturers make many claims pertaining to these products. Some of these are true, some are not. Some are impossible to prove or disprove at this point. For example, if someone claims that a certain product will make us live longer, who's going to know if that's true or not until we're all gone? Some supplements work because of a specific scientific principle, some work purely on a placebo effect, and in some cases it isn't clear at all. Glucosamine and chondroitin sulfate fall into this latter category (see Chapter 5). In any case, people buy nutritional supplements in huge quantities; they buy them out of their own pocket (no insurance pays for this), and if they feel better from the placebo effect, so be it.

Real medicine versus placebos

How does the FDA protect us from placebos? It demands controlled clinical trials. One group of patients gets the new medication while another group gets a pill that looks the same but made of a (presumably) inert substance. Ideally, the study is double blind: neither the doctor nor the patient knows whether he or she is getting the medication or the placebo. They just know it as A or B. After a period of time, the code is revealed. Everyone then knows who got what, and the effectiveness of the medication can be compared to that of the placebo. In fact, that's how people discovered that placebos work! Because even in the placebo group people got better!

In order for a medication to be approved by the FDA it has to be deemed safe (though no medication is 100 percent safe) and it has to work better than a placebo. Is a 30 percent success rate good enough for the FDA? If a placebo works on 2 percent of subjects, the answer is yes. If, however, a placebo was found to work on 29 percent of patients tested the answer is no! When it comes to pain, that's the success rate that we're talking about. So if 30 percent of your friends who've tried this new natural pain medication tell you they love it, they're just getting a placebo effect. *But don't tell them*, you'll ruin it for them.

Placebos über alles?

It is not terribly surprising to find that a placebo alleviates pain. Pain is not a monolithic entity. It's more like a layered cake. There's the actual pain and there is the anxiety associated with it. In some cases the anxiety component is by far the major factor, and it's easy to see how the power of suggestion could address this. I find this all the time when giving injections. Some people clench their fists, break out into a sweat, and cry for their mother at the mere mention of an injection, while others coolly file their nails.

It is harder to imagine how a placebo affects conditions seemingly unrelated to anxiety. The chest pain you get from shoveling snow is due to a lack of oxygen to your heart and is called angina. Parkinson's is a degenerative condition of certain brain cells that can lead to stiffness and tremors. Colitis is an inflammation of the colon. Asthma is a constriction of the air ducts in the lungs. Warts are nasty growths. None of these conditions should be amenable to a placebo, yet all have been found to be (albeit to a certain extent). Where does it end?

Unfortunately, people still get sick and die even when they fervently believe. Cancer is an area that has not been vanquished by placebos. It is therefore a dangerous area to fool around in. The same holds for bacterial infections. People used to die from what today would be called simple infections. Appendicitis was a killer. (Even Houdini could not escape.) If you develop a bacterial infection you want an *evidence-based* medication.

A little respect

What then should be organized medicine's stand on placebos? Once upon a time, placebos, these "lies that heal," were just about the *only* form of treatment available. Though they could not cure cancer nor arrows through the heart, they helped a large number of patients afflicted with a remarkable array of conditions. No one questioned the doctor about his treatment. He was above reproach (there were no shes then). Everyone knew that the doctor's cure rate was limited, but any chance of success lay greatly in belief.

Society has now turned 180 degrees. We expect victory and want no part of any phoney-baloney. The doctor has been stripped of mystery and magic. Instead of the haughty, paternalistic physician who looks down his nose through those little glasses and *tells* you you'll get better, you have the kinder, gentler doctor who tells you about all the terrible things than can go wrong. We are winning the battle over conditions that require science and losing out on those that just need a little placebo. Doctors no longer dare be paternalistic. Society does not accept this.

If a treatment is no better than a placebo, it is reasonable to abandon the treatment, especially if it is expensive or risky. But how about adopting the placebo as the formal treatment? We have arrived at an interesting point in our medical advances: we understand that diseases all have a scientific basis and we have developed scientific treatments for many of these conditions. Many, not all.

Maybe we should take a more scientific look at placebos.

The Reverse Placebo

As noted above, a patient who overly worries about failure and complications is setting him/herself up for a poor result.

On a related note, patients given a diagnosis of a herniated disc, a torn rotator cuff, a torn ligament, a torn meniscus, a torn *anything* will think of themselves as wounded. This messes with their mind: they baby themselves; they can't do this; they can't do that. This protective behavior can on occasion be appropriate; but when the tear or herniation is but an MRI finding with no clinical relevance, the MRI report without appropriate counseling has been harmful to the patient.

CHAPTER 10

Injuring Your Knee in the Name of Health

Summary Soundbite:

Not all exercise equates to health.

Chances are that you exercise. You do so because it's fun, or because you want to keep your weight down, or because it's a way to stay in touch with people, or because everyone else is, or because your doctor told you to do so, or because you feel it will keep you healthy.

These are all good reasons to exercise. However, not all forms of exercise are good for your knee. And it's one thing to injure your knee while having fun, it's quite another to hurt it while going through some tedious routine because it is good for you.

Generally speaking, there are two ways you can hurt your knee: by way of a sudden event or via repetitive use. The former is easy to understand: if you stress the bones, ligaments, tendons, or cartilage beyond a certain point, they will fail. The repetitive injury is more subtle. You can't trace the pain back to any one single event. You're not even sure that your athletic activity triggered the symptoms, but your sport aggravates the pain. Some repetitive injuries are the result of overuse, that is, you've simply done more than what your body can tolerate. You can occasionally overcome this through training, but other times you've simply pushed your envelope as far as it will go. Other repetitive injuries are the result of faulty techniques or equipment, and these should be easier to address. Let us look at some athletic activities.

Running

Running (or jogging) has arguably been the sport most affected by the fitness ardor of the last forty years. Initially, there was concern among sports medicine doctors that pounding on the knee, mile after mile, would lead to early arthritis among running enthusiasts. This fear has not materialized. A healthy, well-aligned knee appears to tolerate running quite well. Of course, we do not yet know the fifty-year effects of repeated, prolonged running, but results so far are encouraging.

And yet, some vigilance is warranted. Note that I stated that a well-aligned knee appears to tolerate running. People who are bow-legged or knock-kneed are at risk for arthritis in the first place because they tend to place all their weight on just one part of the knee. Although there is as yet no conclusive proof of this, it stands to reason that such people may be at even greater risk of arthritis with years of repetitive jogging. I do not recommend jogging to my bow-legged and knock-kneed patients.

Tendinitis (see runner's knee page 134). As the knee bends and straightens, a thick band of tissue running along the outside of the thigh rubs back and forth along the side of the femur (thighbone). This band is called the iliotibial (ITB) band because it starts high up on the ilium (one of the pelvic bones) and runs along the thigh all the way down to the tibia (shinbone). In some people, the repetitive rubbing eventually leads to inflammation and pain. Because the pain is localized to the outside part of the knee joint, the unwary practitioner may suggest that you have "torn cartilage." As we have stated a few times already in this book, this misdiagnosis is even more likely if you have had the misfortune of undergoing an MRI. In the old days, if a patient said, "It hurts when I do this," the doctor's obvious retort was, "Well, don't do this!" That is no longer acceptable. A sports medicine doctor's goal is to get his or her patients back to the activities they love. Nevertheless, part of your treatment will involve cutting back temporarily on your mileage. Stretching, cold packs, anti-inflammatory medications, perhaps physical therapy and injections will be included in the treatment package, after which you can gradually begin to increase your mileage (see Chapter 11).

You should evaluate your running routine. Are you increasing your mileage too rapidly? A 10 percent increase per week has been regarded as a maximum, but for you, even this might be too much. Everybody is different. Listen to your body rather than blindly obey a formula. Are you running on concrete? Of course, you may not have much of choice, but rock-hard surfaces are obviously going to be toughest on your knees. Are you running on hills? Hills are problematic whether you are running up, down, or sideways. Running up or down puts stress on your kneecap, and it puts you at risk for developing pain in the patellofemoral (kneecap) joint. Running sideways on a hill puts your feet and legs at an unnatural angle, and it predisposes you to having pain anywhere from your back down to your feet.

Shoe wear is critical. The running shoe is designed to absorb shock as the foot strikes the ground. It is also designed to support the delicate and intricate mechanism of foot mechanics—the complex interaction of the many bones and ligaments inside the foot during weight-bearing activities. Without a good shoe, the ligaments in the foot would begin to stretch painfully after prolonged running, and the repeated pounding would cause added inflammation. Therefore, a cardinal rule is to check that your shoes are in good condition.

Are you flatfooted? You look under your foot, you see an arch, and you say, "No." Sorry, that's not how to tell. Unless you are severely flatfooted, the arch looks fine until you stand and put all your weight on the foot. Normally, the arch does not touch the ground. (Check out footprints in the sand.) If you are flatfooted, it will. An approximate synonym for flat feet is foot pronation, as in "the foot pronates abnormally." Many scientific (and pseudo-scientific) articles have been devoted to the effect of abnormal foot mechanics on knee pain. Although there still exists controversy as to just how altered foot mechanics can cause knee pain, there is no question that the correlation exists. If your feet are flat when you run, you are at increased risk of developing knee pain. Presumably, your foot twists as it strikes the ground, and this twist gets transmitted up the leg. This then generates painfully abnormal stresses about the knee. That is as specific as I can get without wading into unsubstantiated theories.

Most running shoes have a built-in arch support. This is in contradistinction to the traditional sneakers where the insole is completely flat. Therefore, for most runners, a regular running shoe will suffice. Even an arch that is slightly flat will be adequately supported by the insole of a running shoe. If, however, your foot is very flat, the insole of your running shoe will not suffice. You may need a full-length orthotic. This is an insert that is slipped into your shoe. Such a device will support the arch, restore more normal foot mechanics, and hopefully minimize knee pain.

Though flat feet represent the most common foot abnormality, there are many other variations of foot anatomy that can all potentially predispose to pain. If your foot looks funny in any way, and your knee hurts when you run, consider obtaining an orthopedic or a podiatric consultation. You may benefit from an orthotic in your running shoe.

At the Gym

"I go to the gym" is the answer most people give when I ask whether they exercise. Of all the athletic activities available out there, gym exercises are the ones most likely to be performed strictly for health. Going to the gym represents a commitment to stay or become fit. Although clearly there can be a social aspect, few people go to the gym for fun. It is therefore particularly vexing to get injured at the gym, for this is the ultimate example of injuring yourself in the name of health.

Sudden injuries are incurred when the knee is simultaneously (and rapidly) bent and twisted, as when going from a jump to a squat while turning the torso. The meniscus can pop and require surgery. The same can happen if you get up suddenly from an awkward position. If you suffer from kneecap malalignment, the kneecap can slip out of its groove when you plant your foot and twist your upper body. Turning (with the feet planted on the ground) to throw a basketball is an example of such an activity. You should avoid it if you've ever been told that your kneecap went out or that your patella subluxed, or that your patella dislocated. If you're into lifting weights, you can rupture the patellar tendon while jerking weights that are too heavy for you. This injury will also require surgery and will be associated with a lengthy rehabilitation period. Lunging activities can cause a pulled muscle in the calf or thigh. This is an actual tear of muscle fibers. It is associated with sudden pain, swelling, and discoloration of the skin over a period of a few days. To a certain extent, stretching prior to exercising can prevent muscle pulls. To obtain maximal benefit from stretching, the stretch must be maintained twenty seconds.

Most knee injuries at the gym are related to overuse, that is, excessive repetition of flexion/extension (bending/straightening). Overuse is the medical term for overdoing it. As can happen with running, a knee that is repeatedly bent and straightened is prone to developing tendinitis. If you go through a stair or step routine you may develop pain pertaining to your kneecap. These injuries are relatively easy to treat to the extent that they require simple analgesics, anti-inflammatory medications, ice, and activity modification.

Racket Sports

All racket sports involve considerable bending and twisting from the torso on down. Although tennis elbow, by virtue of its appellation, would seem to be the most common tennis injury, knee pain can't be far behind. Once again, overuse is the major culprit. The weekend warrior syndrome brings people into the office Monday mornings. Players are sore from having simply overdone it. The pain can be just about anywhere about the knee, and the error here is for the doctor to start sending the tennis player for an MRI (unless one or the other is looking for surgery). Barring a sudden injury, the problem is not likely to be a meniscus, despite the inevitable torn cartilage on the MRI report.

Sudden knee injuries are rare in racket sports, although an awkward twist can certainly pop a meniscus or strain a ligament. Also, planting the foot and turning the body is *de rigueur* in these sports, and the kneecap can slip out of its groove in people with a predisposition to this problem. The best way to prevent these injuries is to play on surfaces with some give, such as clay-like surfaces. By allowing the foot to swivel, torque at the knee level is minimized. Common over-the-counter braces, on the other hand, are not likely to prevent an injury. Nevertheless, some players feel more secure with an elastic support around the knee, in which case I give my blessing to its use.

Basketball

Anyone who plays basketball probably reads the sports pages and therefore understands how often basketball players injure their knees. Although ankle sprains are probably more common, knee injuries tend to be more serious.

That serious knee injuries should occur commonly in this sport is hardly a surprise. Lunging, jumping, and landing awkwardly are part and parcel of the game. The accidents incurred span the entire gamut of available injuries: medial collateral ligament (MCL) sprains, anterior cruciate ligament (ACL) and posterior cruciate ligament (PCL) tears, meniscal tears, and kneecap dislocations. Not to mention combinations of the above. The terrible triad is a particularly pernicious combination of an MCL, ACL, and medial meniscal tear.

As any college or professional player will tell you, there is no way to completely prevent these injuries, though it never hurts to be in shape. The heavier you are, the more torque is applied to your knee when you land from a jump.

Women are far more likely than their male counterparts to sustain ACL tears (see Chapter 4). Though the reasons for this are still subject to debate, the fact that a major discrepancy exists between the sexes is not. According to one of the more prevalent theories, women tend to land from a jump in a more stiff-legged manner. This is quite an optimistic hypothesis because the problem should be amenable to training. And the very preliminary results are encouraging: centers that have focused on jumping and landing skills have noted a decrease in women's ligament injuries. This is still a young field, however, and many questions remain unanswered.

"Jumper's knee" is particular to basketball. Pain develops toward the front of the knee as a result of repeated jumping. The pain is caused by an inflammation of the patellar tendon that connects the kneecap to the shinbone (tibia). Though less worrisome than the injuries listed above, it can nonetheless be a stubborn condition. The treatment is standard fare for tendon inflammations: rest (yuk), ice, and anti-inflammatory medications. On rare occasion, chronically abnormal tissue forms within the tendon, and this can require surgery.

Soccer (Football)

With regard to the knee, soccer is similar to basketball. One leg has to be planted while the other kicks, and on the side that is planted, the knee is subject to major twisting forces. Moreover, players are constantly sliding into each other. Thus, all the injuries described for basketball are also common in soccer. Once again, women are even more at risk. Stretching, conditioning, and keeping one's weight down all improve the odds against serious injury, but soccer remains a high-risk activity with regard to the knee.

Golf

How bad for the knees can golf be? There's no running or jumping. And yet. If you consider golf to be a sport and you carry or pull your clubs around the course, there is the obvious stress on the knees associated with lugging a dead weight around for a few miles. As far as your knees are concerned, you just put on an awful amount of weight. If you consider golf more a skill than a sport and you navigate the course in a golf cart, this is obviously milder on the knees. But the golf swing still involves twisting. Depending on the exact nature of your knee condition this may or may not present a problem. For example, if you have a torn meniscus (torn cartilage) the twisting motion of the knee may tug on the tear, and this can be painful. The tear only has to be a fraction of an inch to the right or to the left for this same motion to be painless. The same holds for arthritis. If it's in just the wrong spot the pain of wear and tear can be exacerbated by a golf swing.

With both a torn cartilage and arthritis you are not harming yourself by playing golf—just causing more pain. Consider taking some pain medication just before playing a round (e.g., a combination of an anti-inflammatory medication if your doctor allows it and some acetaminophen).

If your kneecap tends to slip in and out (see Chapter 6) the golf swing can put your kneecap at risk. You would have discovered this early in your golf career. In this situation bracing of the knee can be helpful. (You would need a so-called patellofemoral knee support.)

Skiing

Ski injuries can be minimized by training and by proper maintenance of equipment. In the typical ski injury, the tip of the ski gets caught; the ski veers off to the side while the other ski continues to point straight ahead. Pop goes the medial collateral ligament (MCL) of the knee that's veering off. The better the skier, the less likely this injury is to occur. The anterior cruciate ligament (ACL) is also at risk during skiing. According to a University of Vermont study, among recreational skiers, this injury is most likely to occur when the skier allows him or herself to fall back in a sitting, "hip-below-knee" position. If in addition one ski diverges away from the other, the conditions are right for an ACL tear. Again, the more advanced the skier, the less likely this is to happen.

Slow twisting injuries of the kind sustained in heavy, spring-like snow can also wreak havoc on a knee, as bindings are less likely to release in these conditions.

Fortunately, releasing under a greater variety of conditions than in the past, ski bindings continues to improve. Given a choice, spend the extra money on bindings rather than on skis. On a more negative note, ski boots are higher and more rigid than those of bygone years, and torque is transmitted higher up the leg: boot-top fractures of the shinbone (tibia) have given way to ligament injuries about the knee.

Collisions between skiers remain a danger against which expertise and equipment are powerless. A number of resorts monitor overcrowding and take steps to control speeding.

Snowboarding

With both feet attached to one large board, the snowboarder does not have to worry about one leg veering off in a crazy direction. He or she is therefore relatively immune to the MCL sprain and to the ACL tear. No, snowboarders are more at risk for arm injuries, having no poles to compensate for a loss of balance.

Cycling

Because repetitive bending and straightening of the knee is inherent to the sport, overuse syndromes such as iliotibial (ITB) tendinitis are common. Moreover, the knee can be excessively stressed if a foot which naturally turns in or out is forced by the toe clips to point forward.

Wrestling

The wrestler can injure his medial collateral ligament (MCL), anterior cruciate ligament (ACL), or meniscus, as can any athlete who awkwardly twists his knee. In addition, the wrestler commonly lands directly on his knee, and such trauma can lead to bursitis. If the swelling and pain are mild, no specific treatment is required. On the other hand, severe pain and swelling mandate an aspiration: placement of a needle into the swollen bursa with removal of the fluid.

CHAPTER 11
Exercises for a Healthy Knee

Summary Soundbite

Stretch, Strength, Balance

Treatment protocols for just about any knee condition should incorporate knee exercises. The right knee exercises. This is true whether you are trying to treat a certain condition or trying to prevent it.

Knee exercises can be part of a head-to-toe "stay-in-shape" training program or they can be the sole focus of an exercise session. Either way, they should make you feel good. They are not designed to be a form of torture. Ideally, they should be fun.

So turn on the TV, put on some dance music, and start working those knees!

An exercise program can be divided into categories:

- The aerobic warm-up
- Stretching
- Strengthening
- Balance
- Conditioning
- Water exercises

Step 1. Light Aerobics: Stretching of the shoulders and back

Start the juices flowing with some basic calisthenics. This gets your body and soul into an exercise frame of mind. Run lightly in place. Hold a three- to five-pound weight in each hand. Slowly raise your arms as high as they go ("reach for the sky"). As you strain to reach up, you should feel those tissues about the shoulders stretching, stretching, stretching (See Figure 11-1).

Now as you bring your arms down bring your shoulders way back, military style. Keep running in place. Put the weights down. Grab the back of each shoulder with the opposite hand (See Figures 11-2 and 11-3). Inch your fingers further and further back. Without turning your feet turn your torso all the way to the right and then all the way to the left.

Repeat.

After five minutes of this you are ready to address the knee.

Note: you should be able to comfortably carry on a conversation while running. If not, stop. If your knee hurts, perform the shoulder and back stretches without running.

A basic exercise principle is "warm up, ice down." That is, if it's cold and you feel particularly stiff, warm up. Literally. If the air temperature is cool, wear warm clothing. Discard layers as you work up a light sweat. Consider applying heat directly to a stiff area by way of a warm gel pack. When you are done exercising, ice down the areas that you know will be sore. Cold reduces swelling and acts as a painkiller without side effects. If you are using ice, do not apply it directly on the skin, but rather on a thin towel or cloth. Otherwise, you can get frostbite.

Aerobic tips:

- If the temperature is cool, start by wearing a sweat suit.
- As you work up a light sweat, discard the suit.

- Shoes should be light and supple. (Shoes designed for basketball are designed to resist high levels of torque. Such support is not necessary here, though it is not harmful.)
- When possible exercise in a cool, well-ventilated area. There is no benefit to profuse perspiration.

Step 2. Stretching

Stretching is a key component of any knee program (See Figures 11-1 through 11-9).

I know; it's boring. But yes, it's that important.

Stiffness of any muscle group hampers the normal free-flowing motion of the knee. This slight alteration of muscle tone invisible to the naked eye adds pressure to parts of the knee and can exacerbate existing pain.

And it's not just the muscles that need stretching. The tendons (connecting muscles to bones) also need to get into the act. From a distance they look like ropes. Under a powerful microscope, however, one notes that they consist of millions of little biological springs. With sustained stretching, these miniature springlets uncoil somewhat, and the tendons become a little more elastic. Instead of looking like ropes, these tendons start to behave like rubber bands. The operative word here is sustained. Bouncing around doesn't stretch anything. When you perform a stretching exercise, you must hold that position for twenty seconds. Those little coils don't just unwind at the snap of a finger.

Anatomically, the muscles that control the knee start high up on the leg in the area of hip and pelvis. For example, the hamstrings at the back of the thigh take their origin on the so-called ischial tuberosity, the bone you sit on! One of the muscles that extends your knee (the rectus femoris) starts at the front of your abdomen, just below the belt line. At the other end of the leg, the calf muscles that raise your heels off the ground also bend the knee. In short, one way or the other, just about every muscle in the leg affects your knee.

Stretching exercises for the knee therefore involve the whole leg.

Following an injury or surgery, your knee will not want to straighten all the way. And it will not want to bend. Indeed, bending or straightening puts the ligaments and tendons on stretch, and this is painful. If you give in to the knee's reluctance to straighten and bend, two things may happen: your knee pain may persist or worsen; moreover, you might permanently lose knee motion. "Move it or lose it."

Home exercises

A therapist can't be with you all day long, so you need to exercise on your own too. Figures 11-4 through 11-8 cover basic stretches. Note that with age, the adductors (Figure 11-7) become tight (that's why you have more trouble reaching that tennis ball), and they need to be included in your stretching program.

<u>Trick of the trade:</u> If you have trouble straightening the knee after surgery or after an injury, try this trick (Figure 11-9). Lie on your bed, face down. Wiggle down to the end of the bed until the knee rests right at the edge of the bed. Then just let your leg hang down. The weight of your leg will gradually straighten out the knee. If that doesn't work well enough, put a book or two in a handbag, and let the handbag hang from your ankle. Progressively add books until you feel a difference. By the way, this book has been scientifically designed to be the ideal weight. It's even more effective when you use four at once. (Just kidding.)

Keep in mind that at no point should you experience pain. As with all stretching, give the exercise time. You have to be patient.

<u>How to (and not to) stretch.</u> Watch folks on the tennis court: they lean right, they lean left, now forward, now backward, a little twist here, a little twist there—a waste of time. HOLD THAT STRETCH. With each stretch, you have to count to twenty. Think of the tiny springlets in those tendons. It takes a sustained effort to stretch them out.

Step 3. Strengthening

Weak muscles contribute to wobbly, painful knees. To a certain extent then, strengthening exercises can alleviate pain. But be careful! Certain exercises can themselves be painful. Such exercises are to be avoided! It is not "no pain, no gain."

Strengthening exercises are divided into maintenance exercises and activity-specific exercises. Maintenance exercises provide general fitness. Activity-specific exercises are geared toward training for a specific endeavor.

If you're going to strengthen your knee, you need to work on all the muscle groups discussed above (quadriceps, hamstrings, etc.).

The four quadriceps muscles are at the front of the thigh. They straighten the knee when it is bent, as when, for example, you want to kick a ball. When you stand and your knees are slightly bent (which is most of the time), the quads are the muscles that keep your knee from bending all the way and collapsing. To strengthen your quadriceps, try this exercise: Wrap a two- or three-pound ankle weight to your lower leg and sit on a chair. Straighten the knee slowly and then let your foot down. Repeat a total of ten times. Wait a few moments and repeat. Boring? You bet. Listen to some music or watch a movie. If this exercise is too easy, increase the weight. What, you don't have ankle weights? Time to pull out that handbag again.

Caution: increase weights very gradually. The length of your leg magnifies the effect of the weights at the level of your knee (remember levers in high school?). An increase of just one pound can translate to quite a bit more at the knee.

This exercise is called a leg extension (see Figure 11-10). As long as it does not hurt, it is safe and it is easy. You can certainly do this on your own at home.

Steps—either up or down—are another way to strengthen the quads. Step exercises are a little less practical if you live in a ranch-style house or in an apartment, but in medical lingo they are more "physiological" than leg extension exercises. This means that they approximate everyday activities more closely.

There are pitfalls with every exercise, and step exercises are no exception: the steps should not be too big. The stairs in your house or your apartment building are probably fine, but in some gyms and exercise classes you will only find large step stools. Those might be OK for you, but make sure you can handle normal steps (stairs) first.

Be careful with wall slides! To perform a wall slide, you stand with your back to a wall with your heels a foot or so away from the wall. You gradually slide down and get back up. The further your feet are from the wall, the tougher the exercise. It does strengthen the quads, but it puts a great deal of pressure on your kneecaps. If your kneecaps are fine, you might get away with it, but I don't think it's a very healthy exercise unless you limit how far down you go.

The hamstrings consist of three muscles at the back of the thigh. They serve principally to bend the knee. To strengthen the hamstrings you need ankle weights. Lie on your stomach, and slowly bend the knees. As with leg extensions, gradually increase the weights (gradually).

Perhaps you're thinking that you don't need your hamstrings. (Buzzer) Wrong. Muscle actions about the knee are more complicated than simple bending and straightening. They all work in concert during every activity. More on that below.

The abductors are the muscles on the outer aspect of your thighs. Guess what they do. They abduct the leg! Translation: they swing the leg away from the body. When you are standing, the abductors raise the leg off to the side. A (male) dog abducts his leg at the fire hydrant. You can strengthen these muscles by standing with ankle weights on, abducting your leg slowly, and letting it back down—another exciting exercise. (There's a reason for all that music in exercise classes.)

The adductors live on the inner aspect of your thigh and have the opposite function. They bring the leg in line with your body. That happens naturally when you're standing, but if you're lying down with your leg out (say you're doing an abduction exercise), it's the adductors that bring the leg back in. Strengthening the adductors is a little more involved because, by and large, gravity does their work. As soon as you lift your leg (abduct) to the side, gravity will work against the abductor muscles to bring the leg back down. So, to strengthen the adductors, stand with a heavy object between your feet and try to push it toward the other foot. Push for ten seconds and relax. Repeat until bored. That's likely to be about five seconds. So actually give yourself a target of ten repetitions and move on to another exercise (for example, strengthening the abductors of the other leg).

Wide elastic bands can substitute for weights and are commercially available (e.g., Theraband®). They come in different colors, each representing a certain resistance. You tie one end of the band around your ankle and the other end around the foot of a table. Pull your foot away from the table, and you're working your adductors (See Figure 11-12). If you've gone ahead and bought these bands, you might as well use them for other exercises. Sit on a chair facing a table. In fact, sit with your leg straight out as far from the table as the elastic band allows. Now bend the knee. The elastic band will offer resistance, and you will be working your hamstrings. Now, instead of tying one end of the band around a table, tie it around the foot of your chair. When you straighten your knee, the elastic band will once again offer resistance, and you will be working your quads.

Step 4. Balance

One of the world's most famous basketball players consulted one of the world's foremost spine surgeons. This world-class athlete had been told of a disc herniation and had been advised to consider surgery. The surgeon found that his patient could not stand on one leg with his eyes closed. He required no surgery.

No matter how fit, how trim, how muscular, how coordinated, or how talented you are, your balance can be poor. And it will get worse with age. The good news is that you can work on your balance just as you do your strength. For starters, stand on one leg thirty seconds, then the other; then do so with your hip bent at a right angle (knee level with your hip); then do so with your eyes closed; then do so with your arms stretched out in front of you.

To facilitate these exercises, check out an app called Gyrobalance.

Balance exercises teach your muscles to work in a coordinated fashion (with thanks to Jean-Pierre Farcy, MD).

Step 5. Conditioning

Conditioning is the practice of getting ready for a particular activity.

There are two aspects of conditioning: building up endurance, and preparing the muscle groups to work with each other.

The concept of endurance is easy to understand. Anyone who has huffed and puffed running for a bus already knows all about it. Your heart, your lungs, your muscles, and every other fiber in your body have to gear up for prolonged activity. You accomplish this by, well, doing it. You start with a short period of exercise and you build up by doing a little more with each exercise session. The common wisdom is that you should be able to carry out a conversation while exercising. If you're so out of breath that you can't talk, stop.

The concept of preparing muscle groups to work together is less intuitive. Think of super-strong men with powerful weapons. As strong as they may be, collectively they would not make a great army their first day on the job. They have to learn to work as a team. They must anticipate the job that needs to be done, and they must move in a coordinated manner to achieve their objectives. The same goes for your knee. Whether you're picking a quarter off the floor, climbing steps, or kicking the winning field goal, all muscles about your knee come into play. Naturally, if you're kicking a ball, the quads may work harder than the hamstrings, but the fact is that even the hamstrings contract. That smooth motion you get when engaging in any activity comes from the seamless interaction of the multiple muscle groups about the knee. That comes with practice.

<u>Feedforward.</u> You've heard of feedback. It's a response to something or someone. Feedforward is anticipation. As the ball

heads your way, your muscles already know what they're going to do. Like a well-trained army, each unit knows its job. The quads will contact just so much, and will do so a split second before such and such muscles and a split second after these others. A moment later they'll relax a bit while the hamstrings kick in. Then you miss your shot, curse, and start again.

Show a pianist the sheet music to *Für Elise*, and the millions of muscle spindles in her forearm will quickly takes their proper place, ready to fire at precisely the right moment. This kind of anticipation only comes with practice. Practicing *Für Elise* that is! Practice Mozart's *Turkish Rondo* instead, and your *Für Elise* will sound like *Fürgetaboutit*. In short, the only way to train for an activity is to mimic it.

Step 6. Water Exercises

Because of gravity, the mere act of standing on land causes pressure on your knees. When you stand in water, chest deep, you are suddenly much lighter. You are said to be more "buoyant." (I sense that you are not surprised.) Exercises that would be too painful on land suddenly become conceivable in water.

What, you don't swim? You don't like to get your head wet? No matter. You can get plenty of exercise in the shallow end of the pool. For starters, have you ever tried *running* in the shallow end of the pool? It's very tiring. It's a "good" tiring too. It's aerobic, meaning that blood is rapidly flowing through the muscles, bearing oxygen and other goodies. It doesn't raise your blood pressure, because you're never straining that hard.

You can lunge forward, you can leap right and left, and you can even perform jumping jacks. The water resists your every movement and strengthens each muscle group.

Providing that the water is warm enough, the pool has a limbering effect. Some of those stretches become a little easier (not the ones where you sit on the ground—avoid doing those in the pool).

This brings us to the point of pool temperature: if the water is too cold, it may actually lead you to stiffen up. So check the temperature before signing up. You might also consider a thin wet suit.

Some physical therapy outfits feature underwater treadmills. I give them the thumbs up.

The deep end of the pool opens up another array of exercises, with or without getting your head wet. A number of arm and leg attachments have been developed to increase the water's resistance as you move about. These are good, as long as you are not overworked. As noted above, in order to insure that you are not overstressing your heart, you should be able to carry out a simple conversation while you exercise. These resistive devices make your muscles work harder and the muscles therefore become stronger.

When planning a vacation, it's not a bad idea to look for places that have a warm pool.

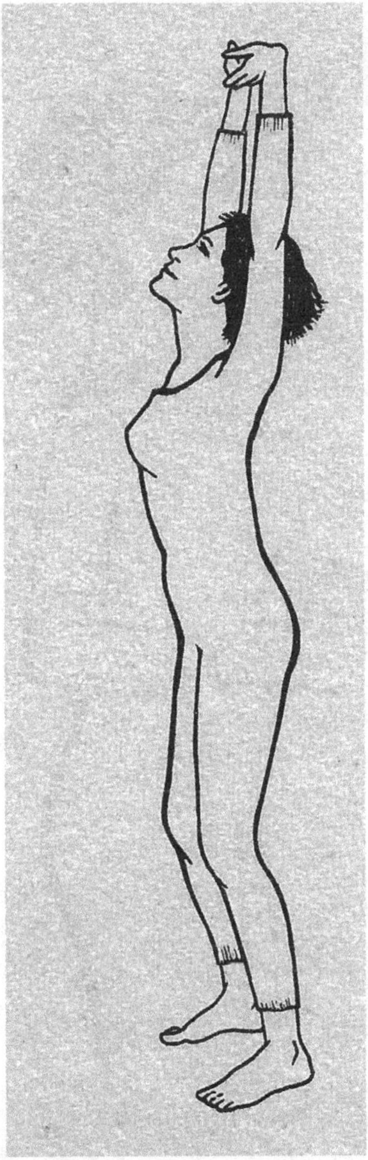

Figure 11-1. Prior to starting knee stretching, it's a good idea to begin with general stretches, e.g. "Reach for the sky."

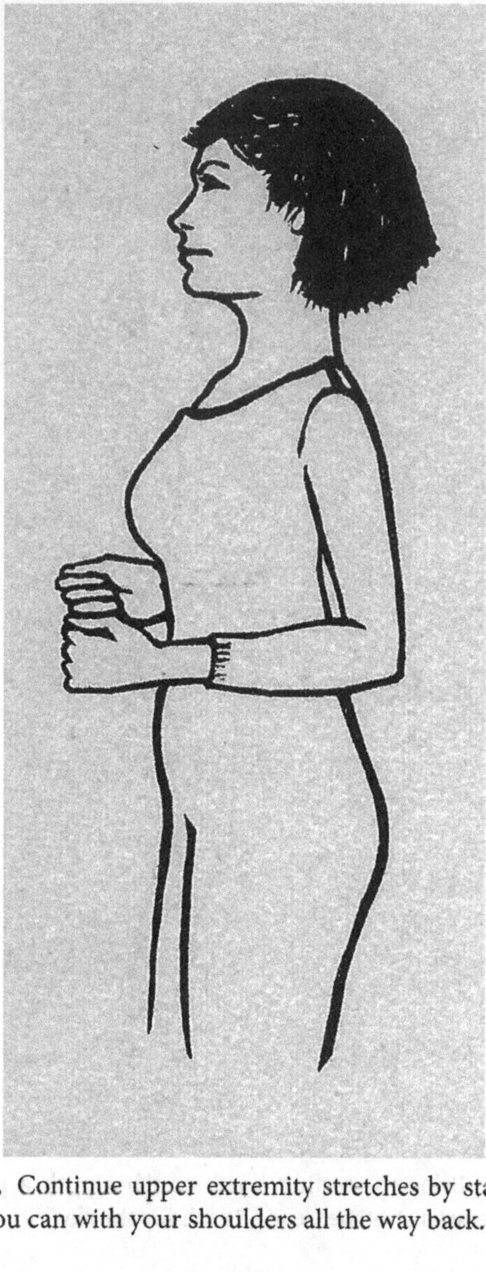

Figure 11-2. Continue upper extremity stretches by standing up as straight as you can with your shoulders all the way back.

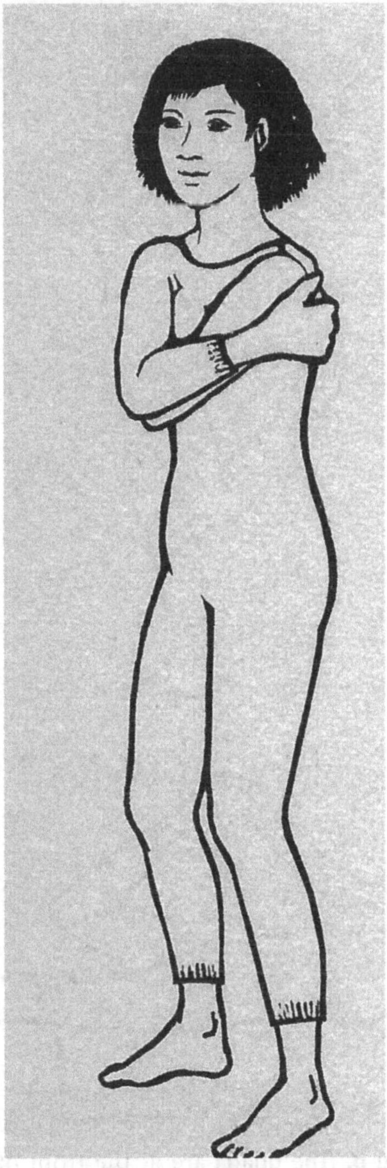

Figure 11-3. More of the same. Reach behind your shoulders as far, far back as you can.

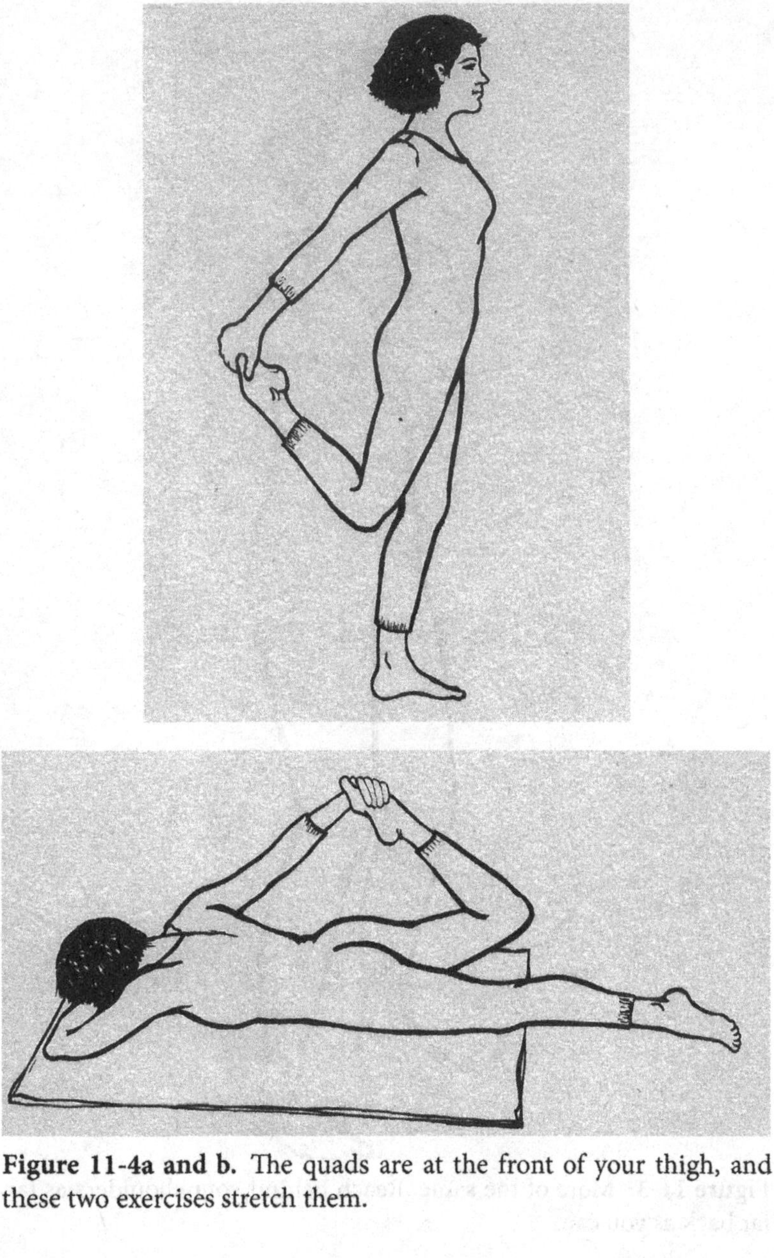

Figure 11-4a and b. The quads are at the front of your thigh, and these two exercises stretch them.

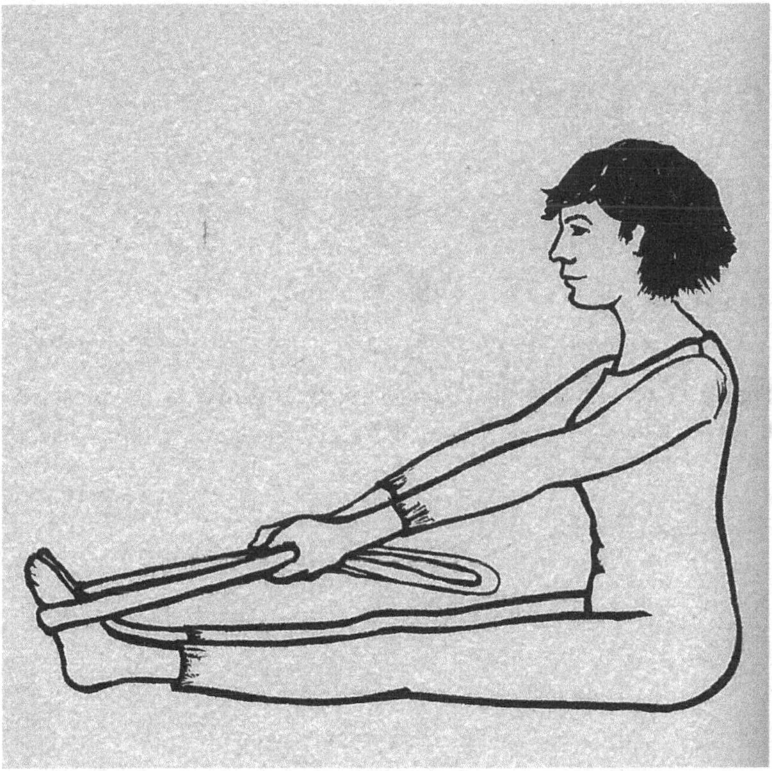

Figure 11-5. Hamstring stretch. (Proceed cautiously if you have any history of low back pain and/or pain shooting down your leg (sciatica).)

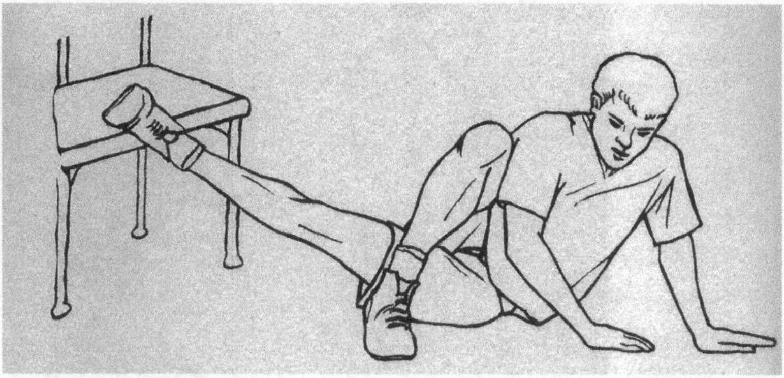

Figure 11-6. ITB (iliotibial band) stretch. This may be the most difficult stretch.

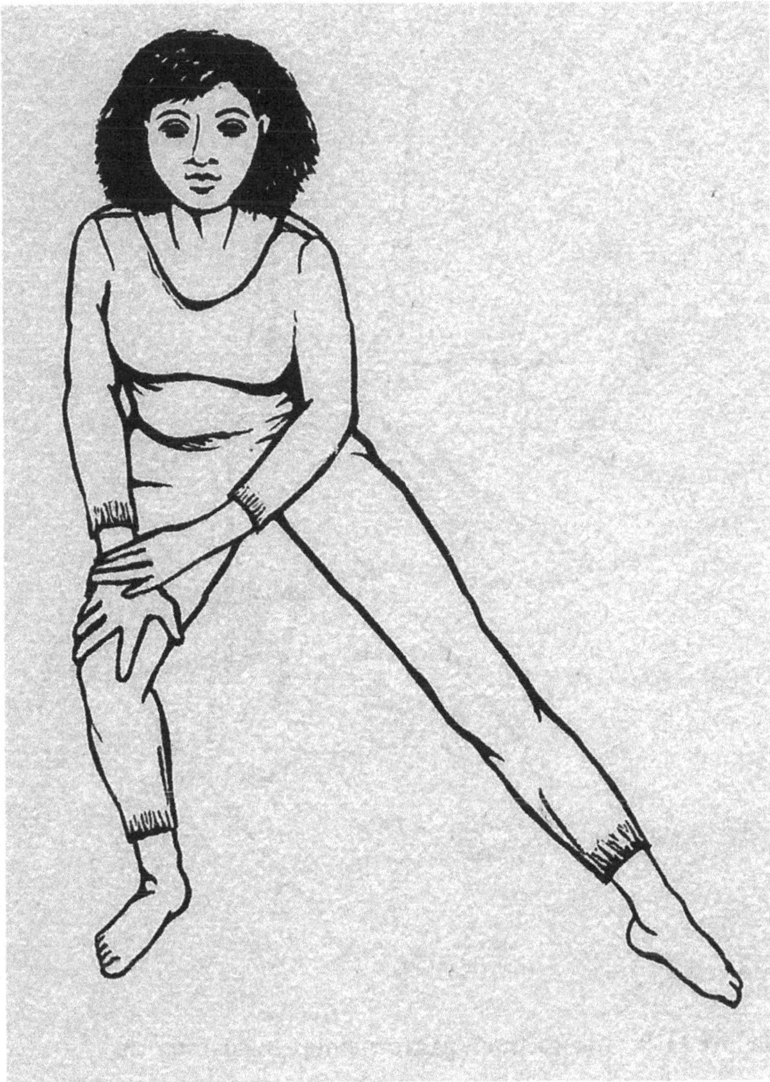

Figure 11-7. The adductor stretch. (The adductor muscles and tendons run along the inner thigh.)

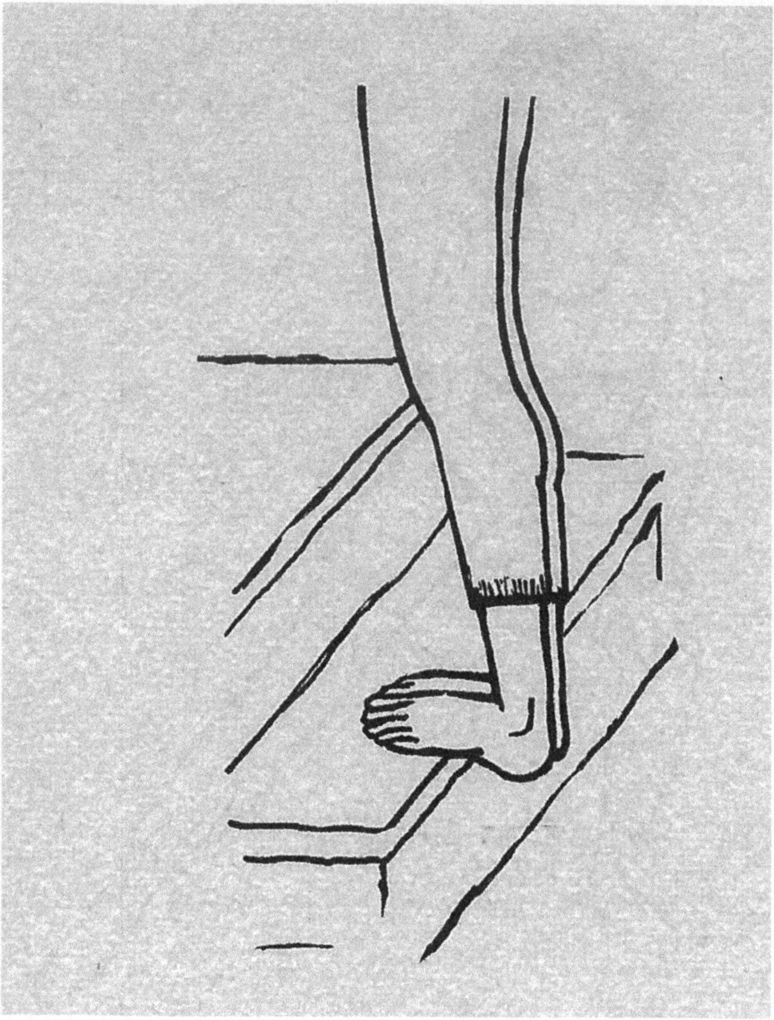

Figure 11-8. The "gastroc" (gastrocnemius-soleus) stretch.

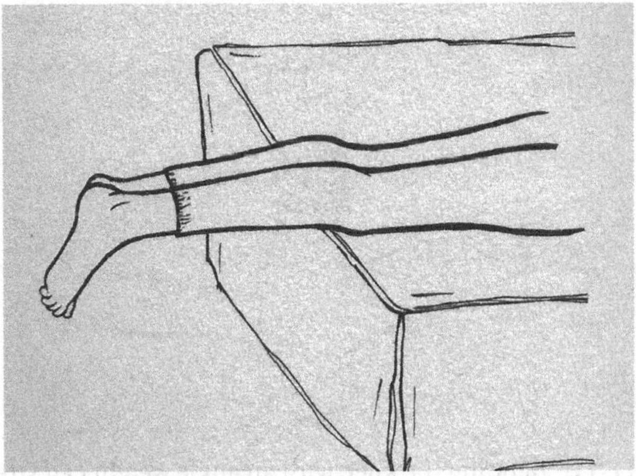

Figure 11-9. Secret "trick of the trade": Stretching a knee that won't straighten after surgery. You can add a *light* ankle weight.

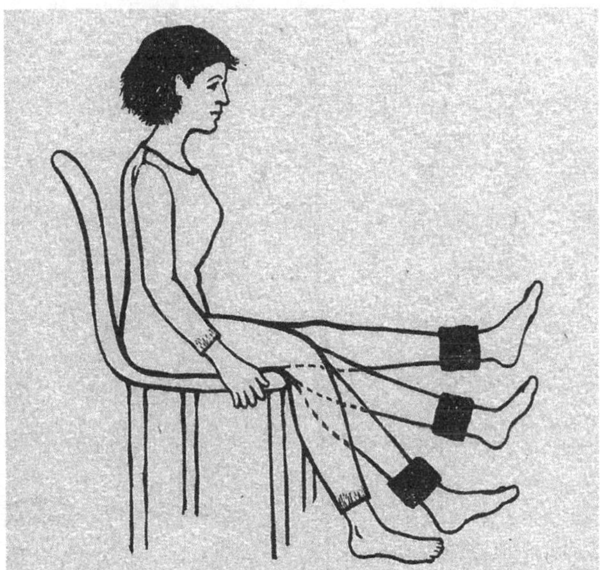

Figure 11-10. Leg extensions. Again, use only light weights. (*The lower leg is a long lever arm that will significantly multiply the effect of the ankle weight.*)

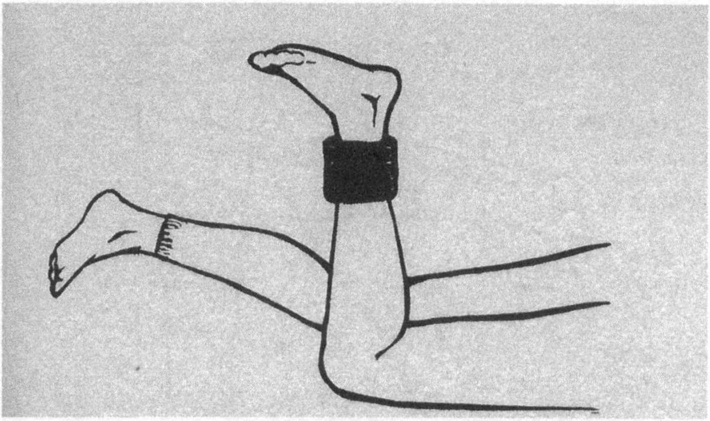

Figure 11-11. Bending the knee with an ankle weight can strengthen the hamstrings.

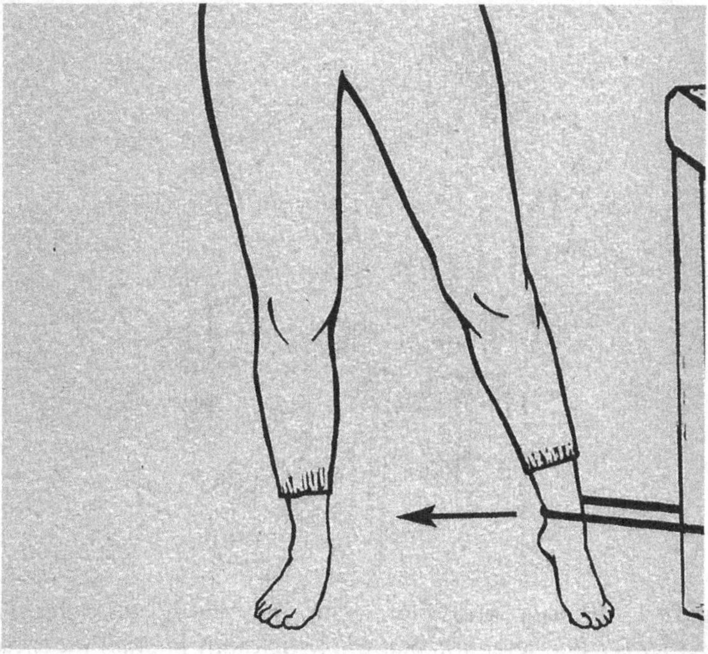

Figure 11-12. Adductor strengthening.

CHAPTER 12
Personal Injury and the Law

> "This world is a comedy to those that think, a tragedy to those that feel."[14]

Your knee hurts as a result of an injury and you've hired a personal injury lawyer. This features a code of ethics that may be different from what you're used to. (Welcome to attorneys who will zoom in to this chapter of the book.)

There is a chance that your lawsuit will be played fairly. Your doctor will prescribe appropriate tests and procedures, he or she will go to bat for you by conveying an honest assessment of your situation, and your lawyer will seek fair compensation for your injury. The other side will consist of an equally honest defendant, an equally honest lawyer, and equally honest doctors. The two sides will square off, like two equally matched teams, and prior to going to trial the two sides will come to an agreement. You will receive fair compensation for your past and future injury-related aggravations.

Unfortunately, this may not happen; there is a chance that one side or the other will be prone to serious denial and/or exaggeration and/or outright fraud.

On the one hand, without knowing anything about you, those who might be financially responsible for your injury occasionally

[14] Horace Walpole, *Letters*. August 16, 1776.

treat you right off the bat as though your claim is dishonest. Admittedly, they see their fair share of cheats. This can lead to a knee-jerk reaction of paying experts to *automatically* say that there is nothing wrong with you (which in any given case might actually be true) regardless of your condition. Or, if they can't dispute the existence of a painful condition, they will *automatically* wave it off as being unrelated to the accident (which can also be true). The key word here is automatically. These doctors aren't simply exercising their constitutional right to voice an opinion. By routinely and automatically voicing the same opinion over and over without regard for the merits of the case, these doctors are perjuring themselves for a fee.

The injured parties' lawyers and their experts are no better. If you go to a busy, honest lawyer, he or she will try to find out the truth and will tell you what your odds are of being compensated, but a lawyer who is not busy and/or dishonest works differently. He may, for instance, send you to three equally unscrupulous doctors: a radiologist who will automatically find a torn cartilage or torn ligament, an orthopedist who will gladly operate on these fictitious injuries and swear that all of your knee problems are due to your injury, and a rehabilitation doctor or chiropractor who will provide months of treatment to back up your claim of severe pain and disability. (The number of injured parties who see a lawyer before seeing a doctor is remarkable.)

A lawyer may focus on the torn meniscus of an MRI report knowing full well that the reading represents a serious (intentional?) over-read. By the same token, he and his doctors may be overlooking more significant conditions such as RSD, a tight iliotibial band, a neuroma, a kneecap problem, etc. (see Chapters 6 and 7).

A variation on this theme occurs when you have a legitimate problem—but the surgeon and lawyer intentionally magnify it far beyond reason. This is another form of dishonesty. The net result is that once the dishonesty is revealed, you take a chance on losing everything. It's akin to stretching a double into an inside-the-park homerun—and getting thrown out at the plate.

The best example of this is arthritis. If you recall from Chapter 5, arthritis is the wearing out of the articular cartilage at the end of your bones. It may or may not be painful. If you are young (or middle-aged), heavy, athletic, bow-legged or knock-kneed, and/or involved in a physical job, your knee arthritis will most likely lead to an eventual knee replacement. Suppose that despite advanced arthritis, your knee doesn't hurt much; you've never seen a doctor for knee pain. One day you fall onto your knee and it starts to hurt. Your doctor and lawyer may honestly claim that the date of your knee replacement was moved up since the accident took a knee that didn't hurt and changed it to a knee that hurt a great deal. A dishonest lawyer, however, will try to pin your knee replacement (and all future knee replacements) on this one fall—ignoring completely the fact that you were going to need this surgery anyway.

The above scenario occurs over and over again and represents an enormous waste of our legal and financial resources.

The party responsible for your injury should recognize that though the need for a knee replacement was not caused by the accident, the date of the replacement was indeed moved up—and plaintiffs' attorneys should stop pretending that their client would never have needed surgery but for the injury.

How much compensation should you receive for having needed knee surgery a few years sooner? That is for society as a whole to decide, not me; however, here is my rule: If 50 percent of Americans would be happy to sustain the injury in exchange for the financial reward, while 50 percent would reject both the injury and the award, then the award is probably about right.

<u>Example:</u> the reward for a wrong-sided knee arthroscopy has been around $400,000. Since I suspect that 95 percent of Americans would gladly undergo an unnecessary arthroscopy for this price (including yours truly), this compensation is far too high.

Beyond serious exaggeration there comes fraud, an example of which is the intentional fabrication on the part of the surgeon of a condition that does not exist and the claim of having performed procedures that never took place.

The motivation is financial.

Fraud in the area of knee pain and surgery is easy and more common than you'd like to think. (Much of what I say about knees can be transposed to other parts of the body.)

Creating a fraudulent case

Here is how easy it is. (Hopefully none of this will look familiar to you. I thank my dishonest colleagues for making this part of the book possible.)

1. The doctor devotes minimal time to the examination of your knee; he/she doesn't ever examine you while you're standing, let alone walking; it may be appropriate to examine your skin for sensitivity and to place you on your side to test for tightness of the iliotibial band (Chapter 7), but he/she never does that; he doesn't seem to pay much attention to exactly how you hurt your knee; he only obtains two x-ray views rather than four, and you're lying down rather than standing while the x-rays are taken. From visit to visit, the "examination" part of the office notes remains essentially unchanged.
2. The doctor then orders an MRI. This seems perfectly normal to you. (Don't you feel entitled to one?) What you don't know is that regardless of the circumstance, the MRI is likely to indicate a "torn meniscus" (see Chapters 2 and 3). It may well be the very first line of the MRI report even when there are more important findings. (I've often felt as though it's there even before you have the test.)
3 The MRI has now become a license to operate:

   "Gosh, you have a torn meniscus."

   "Gee, could you fix that?"

   "I think we can squeeze you in..."

   There is no attempt on the part of the orthopedist or rehab doctor to see whether your mechanism of injury could possibly have caused a meniscus to tear at the back of the knee. (For example, hitting the dashboard won't cause a meniscus to tear.) In the same spirit, your doctor never seems to wonder what painful condition you could have that won't show up on the MRI (Chapter 7).

4. The surgeon performs the requisite arthroscopy. Depending on her degree of (dis)honesty, she will find one torn meniscus, two torn menisci, an ACL that needs "a little tightening," articular cartilage in need of co-ablation . . . The opportunities are endless for the creatively dishonest surgeon.
5. Either he won't take the requisite intraoperative pictures ("We never take pictures") or the pictures will show just normal tissue, and/or the pictures somehow won't be available for your (or anyone else's) review. ("The hospital must have lost them.")

   In such a case, you are now totally dependent on the honor system, and as we've seen in this book, this is not always an arthroscopist's strong suit.
6. The surgeon generates a report to your attorney indicating "a severe and permanent injury that will require more surgeries." He will opine that your injury is the source of your knee problems (and why not your back and the other knee too?). He will ignore the fact that you'd had knee pains in the past for the same condition (maybe even the recent past).
7. The lawyer plays the ostrich. He's "only going by the doctors' reports" and just wants to help his client.
8. If called upon, the doctor will go to court and swear that there were terrible injuries in need of multiple surgeries, endless therapy, etc...

For emphasis, let me state again that some patients (perhaps you) truly have needed surgery, physical therapy, and the like as a result of a knee injury, and you will want a surgeon who will go to bat for you.

The right to an opinion

An expert is naturally entitled to his or her opinion. However, when that opinion is totally fabricated simply to please someone and is not based on any existing body of knowledge or current thinking, there's a problem. The expert understands perfectly well that he cannot substantiate his opinion, but he'll voice it anyway.

Here are some examples I've encountered:

- A woman claimed that she needed a knee replacement as a result of a car accident; the damage to her car was minimal; by her own admission, her knee never struck any part of the car; she had knee arthritis at the time of the accident and had seen a doctor for this in the past. The "expert" hired by her attorney swore under oath that the mere fact that she'd been shaken up was enough to account for her need for a knee replacement. (Wouldn't everyone on a roller coaster then need a knee replacement?)
- A man fell getting into a bus; he was obese and had been treated over many years for knee pain and arthritis; he'd had prior falls onto his knee that were much more severe than this particular one. Nevertheless, he decided to sue the bus company. His expert opined that in fact this was the particular injury that led to the need for a knee replacement. No particular evidence for this opinion was put forth. It was just his opinion.
- A woman in the back seat of a car alleged that her knee had hit the back of the (padded) seat in front of her. Due to some serious medical conditions at the time, she was on the list for an organ transplant and was being followed very, very carefully by her doctors who carefully listed all (*all*) her medical issues from head to toe at each visit. For many months following the accident they made no note of any knee pain. Suddenly, knee pain. It was her expert's opinion that she'd torn a meniscus at the time of her car accident and now needed surgery.
- A patient sustained a known complication from surgery. This particular complication can be the result of negligence on the part of the surgeon, but is also recognized as occurring when the procedure is carried out "by the book"; unless you were there, it's impossible to tell. The expert stated under oath that he could tell it was negligence.

It works in the other direction too: an expert once testified that a patient of mine with a traumatic saphenous nerve neuritis (Chapter 7) couldn't have anything painful since the MRI was negative. Another "expert" took advantage of an inadequate radiology report to testify that a patient with impressive kneecap issues really had nothing wrong.

The "Consequential" Injury

If some time down the road, say a year or two, your opposite knee starts to hurt, your attorney (with a little assist from your doctor) may claim that this new pain is the result of your "putting more weight" on that leg. This is the "consequential" argument. And while the argument is reasonable in certain cases, by and large it does not apply, as obvious as it may seem. (Many obvious phenomena are actually untrue: the sun does not orbit around the Earth; the Earth is not at the center of the universe, etc . . .)

YOUR LEG CAN'T BEAR MORE THAN THE WEIGHT OF YOUR BODY (unless you're wearing a backpack)! Regardless of whether your left leg hurts or not, the right leg will continue to bear your body weight.

Here's what really happens: if your left leg hurts (foot, knee, hip, . . .) you will take a quick step on the left and spend more time on the right; but spending more time on the right is not going to tear your meniscus or cause you to develop arthritis. You will NOT require surgery as a result of spending more time on that leg. (If you already have arthritis, spending more time on that leg might render the arthritis painful sooner. In this sense, and in this sense only, can an attorney make a "consequential argument.")

The Settlement

Suppose you signed up for a million-dollar winner-take-all tournament. Now imagine being paid $100,000 to drop out ("settle"). The American tradition of the settlement is what makes this process worthwhile to you. You don't have to win. You don't even have to be in the right. Your opponent just has to believe that you *might* win a jury over. Then they pay you to go away. For people who have truly been wronged, it is a reasonable system. For those who are dishonest, it has been an easy scam.

Summary: Our current system is often unfair. Good and bad guys are thrown into a lottery where, to the outsider, payouts appear to be randomly assigned. One person with a minimal injury can win a good settlement if the MRI shows "something," yet doctors miss injuries that will *not* appear on an MRI report, leaving the injured party with no compensation at all. The MRI is both one of the greatest imaging tools around and one of the greatest sources of unwarranted claims.

In a society that prides itself on fair play, it is surprising to me that such a system could still exist. I would favor a system that demands MRI reports that do not mislead, a system requiring doctors to perform a reasonable examination (including a thorough x-ray examination), a system requiring arthroscopy pictures to be taken and made available, a system requiring an expert to offer concrete backing for his or her opinion, and perhaps an arbitration system whereby a panel of knowledgeable people would pass judgment on the merits of injuries.

CHAPTER 13
How to Find the Right Knee Doctor

At this point, you'll want to find a knee doctor who possesses the knowledge and ethics described in this book. For this, you might consult:

- The doctor nearest you.
- The doctor with the most impressive website.
- The doctor referred by a friend or coworker.
- The team doctor for your favorite professional team.
- The doctor referred by your family physician.
- A doctor taken from the list of Board Certified doctors provided by a State Medical Society or by the American Academy of Orthopaedic Surgeons.
- The doctor recommended by a hospital's referral service.
- A doctor listed in "The Best Doctors in (Your City)."
- A doctor referred by a sports medicine (nonsurgical) specialist.
- A doctor referred by a nurse, resident in training, or administrator at a hospital.
- A doctor with an impressive résumé.
- A department Chairman.

- The doctor recommended by your lawyer.
- A doctor referred by another orthopedist.

Each of these has merit, yet one stands out as being better than all others. Let us look at each individually.

The doctor nearest you

Obviously, by simply going to the doctor nearest you, you are taking a major gamble. This requires no explanation.

The doctor with the most impressive website

Most savvy customers will know not to be impressed by an advertisement, since it merely reflects the doctor's willingness to spend money on promotion. Educated customers, though, can still be taken in by websites. It is important to keep in mind that a doctor can make any claim on his or her home page. A health professional can pay to have an entire textbook on the web! It doesn't mean that the health professional actually knows everything in that book or has even read it!

The web is merely the phone book of this millennium.

The doctor referred by a friend or coworker

A doctor recommendation from a friend, relative, or coworker is frequent. Everybody goes to the best doctor in town (ever hear of anybody going to the second-best doctor around?) and people freely dispense advice. Such a recommendation tells you that at least someone has gotten better under that doctor's care—but it doesn't tell you if it was thanks to or in spite of the doctor. It also doesn't tell you about the doctor's ethics or knowledge of your particular problem. The doctor who was great at treating your buddy's back pain may not be so hot when it comes to diagnosing your knee condition. Perhaps at least you can get a sense of whether the doctor is test- and knife-happy.

The team doctor for your favorite professional team

There's a reason why hospitals will dearly pay professional teams to have one of their docs be the Team Orthopedist: being a team doctor is a terrific draw. And nothing is going to change this basic fact of life. The thinking of course is that "if he's good enough for the Jersey Jupiters, he's good enough for me." Having said that, is he really good enough for the Jupiters? Sometimes yes, sometimes no. There are some very knowledgeable and ethical team doctors, and some, well, not so much so. The position of team doctor is not always won on merit.

The doctor referred by your family physician

One thing that can be said for your family physician is that he or she has your best interests in mind—which is a start. Not all family physicians, though, recognize the intricacies of orthopedics to the point of differentiating between orthopedists who are particularly strong in one area versus those who are strong in another area. Ask your doctor whether he or she would recommend the same orthopedist whether you had back or knee pain.

A doctor taken from the list of Board Certified doctors provided by your State Medical Society or by the American Academy of Orthopaedic Surgeons (www.aaos.org)

Board Certification is not a bad thing. If an orthopedist has been certified at some point by the American Board of Orthopedic Surgery, it tells you that the surgeon has studied diligently to pass a written and oral examination. But in the setting of knee pain, Board Certification is not as important as it might seem. The Board Certification examination covers an enormously wide range of subjects including dwarfism, metallurgy, muscle physiology, cartilage biochemistry, wheelchair principles, and prosthetic limbs. (Recertification can be more specific.) Thrown into the examination are a few questions pertaining to the topics in this book. Moreover, Board Certification is no guarantee of honesty, and as we have seen, it is very easy for an orthopedist to pull the wool over someone's eyes. In short, Board Certification by itself is not a good selection criterion.

The doctor recommended by a hospital's referral service

All major hospitals have a referral service, usually with a catchy toll-free telephone number such as 1-877-COM TO US. They will never tell you, "We don't have anyone who does knees." Instead, they'll read you the names of orthopedists who have listed themselves as being interested in knees (or sports medicine or joint reconstruction). This, if you will, is the Yellow Pages® of the hospital and just about as useful. You are better off contacting the orthopedic department directly, though here, the staff will have allegiance to the Chairman and to his or her inner circle.

A doctor listed in a "best of" directory

There are a number of publications purporting to give you a list of the best professionals around. Some are for real and some are bogus. Here's how the bogus ones work. Doctors are sent an application to fill out: name, address, specialty, etc. The doctors who take the time to complete the form are included in the directory. When the book comes out, who buys it? All the doctors listed, of course! Everybody wins: the doctors are listed in a prestigious-sounding text, the publishing company earns a profit from all the doctors who bought the book, and nobody can accuse the doctors of having paid to be listed. Well, almost everybody wins. Anybody leafing through such a book in search of "the best doctors" is rolling the dice.

Other directories make more of an effort to truly find the best doctors. Be aware that these are imperfect too. Some excellent surgeons toil in relative obscurity. They may not publish or lecture much and therefore will remain unknown outside their hospital. Others will have only just recently moved to your area. Yet others are of the shy retiring type and will not attract any attention. This is somewhat rare for orthopedic surgeons. On the other side of the coin, well-connected doctors can occasionally make it into these directories independent of their abilities and ethics.

Read the first pages of any "best doctors" book to see how the doctors were selected. If there is no explanation or only a vague one, you know what you are dealing with.

A doctor referred by a sports medicine (nonsurgical) specialist

A specialty has (relatively) recently emerged called sports medicine. This is very confusing, because a number of medical and surgical specialties like to give themselves this title. The sports medicine I am referring to here is a medical (nonsurgical) specialty dealing with every aspect of athletic medicine, including injury, training, physiology, performance enhancement, management of concomitant medical conditions, etc. In the United States, there are still relatively few such doctors, and their prevalence varies considerably from state to state. They themselves see and treat patients with knee pain, and therefore they are subject to the same issues discussed in the other chapters of this book. In other words, their understanding of the knee may or may not be limited. Although they do not operate and therefore do not have an immediate interest in recommending unnecessary surgery, their financial compensation may in fact be tied to the financial health of their group, and if you need surgery, they will have some obligation to refer you for surgery to someone in that group.

A doctor referred by a nurse, resident in training, or administrator at a hospital

A hospital staff sees knee surgeons up close and personal. But few staff members see all the important aspects of a surgeon's practice. Nurses in the operating room get a sense of a surgeon's speed, but can't say much about bedside manners or a surgeon's indications for surgery. Floor nurses can tell you about bedside manners and post-operative attention to patients, but are less informed on technical ability and again, surgical indications. Administrators can tell you which surgeons are busy, but can't tell you why they are busy. (Are they good doctors or just good salesmen?) Residents (surgeons in training) are a good source of information with regard to the surgeons at their particular hospital, especially if they have a chance to participate in that surgeon's office hours. Because they are in training though, they may lack some perspective and are susceptible to being won over by charismatic surgeons and/or swell guys who let them perform surgery. They also lack the ability to compare their teachers to other surgeons in town.

A doctor with an impressive résumé

An impressive résumé tells you that the surgeon has given a great deal of thought to his/her area of study. If he is asked to lecture, he is probably thought of as being knowledgeable, and more significantly, if he is widely published he probably has expertise in the area of his publications. A résumé, though, doesn't tell you about patient management and ethics.

A department Chairman.

The Chairperson of an orthopedic department is highly ethical, good-looking, intelligent, and highly skilled,[14] and it is natural

[14] My chairperson could conceivably be reading this book.

for patients to seek out the advice of such a doctor. Chairmen are chosen on the basis of their particular expertise in one area of orthopedics and/or leadership and administrative skills. Their appreciation for the subtleties of the knee ranges from excellent to minimal, depending on their area of expertise. Chairmen are usually surrounded by a well-organized staff and have the full attention of the senior orthopedic residents (residents in their last year of training). This may or may not compensate for the fact that some Chairmen are away from their practice a great deal. Make sure this is not something that would bother you.

The doctor recommended by your lawyer

A surprising number of Americans with knee pain see the doctor chosen by their lawyer. This is sometimes reasonable, as when your attorney knows some of the best orthopedists around. Alas, very often a lawyer has a none-too-altruistic ulterior motive: $$$$. Personal injury lawyers who are not completely above board know which radiologists will find something wrong on the MRI and which orthopedists will detect a condition that can only be corrected with months of therapy and surgery. Therefore, if there's nothing really wrong with you and you want to put dollars in your pocket, this is the path to follow. Otherwise, beware.

A doctor referred by another orthopedist

Bingo. A referral from an orthopedist is not easy to come by, unless you happen to be related to one or have one as a friend (everybody should!). Nevertheless, this is your best bet. You might even consider paying for a consultation just to get such a referral. Orthopedists know the orthopedic BSers in their community as well as the guys with suspect ethics. They know this better than any layperson and for obvious reasons, better than doctors in other specialties. The advice of an orthopedist is not foolproof, of course. If you live in a large community, no orthopedist will be familiar with the particular strengths and shortcomings of all his colleagues. Rivalries and jealousies can color an orthopedist's opinion. Conversely, an orthopedist may be interested in returning a favor to a colleague. Nevertheless, it is unlikely that an orthopedist would let you make a big mistake.

In an ideal world, you would have access to all of the above options, and they would all point to one or two knee doctors in your community. Realistically, you will have access to just a few of the options I have listed. My advice would be to use as many as possible.

CHAPTER 14

Should You Have Surgery in an Outpatient Surgical Center?

Outpatient surgical centers ("surgi-centers") are very beneficial to surgeons, insurance carriers, and possibly to you. "Facility fee" is the buzzword. When you undergo a procedure at a facility (hospital or surgi-center), that facility receives a fee from the insurance carrier. Insurance companies pay a surgi-center a lower facility fee than a hospital because the center's expenses are lower. The insurance companies are happy to be paying the lower rate. At the same time, a surgeon who is a part owner of the surgi-center gets a piece of the facility fee, a piece that can be a significant multiple of the surgical fee. The surgeon is happy.

This is all perfectly ethical—assuming that the surgeons are honest with themselves and with their patients.

The benefit to you is that surgi-centers are often more efficient than hospitals meaning that you don't spend as much time waiting; your procedure is more likely to be on time and in theory there may be a lower risk of acquiring infections. (This remains to be fully analyzed and may vary from facility to facility.) In addition, the surgi-center setting will be less crowded and noisy. The waiting room will be quiet and pleasant. Seating may consist of plush armchairs. There may be flowers. It may feel more like an exclusive airport lounge and less like Grand Central Station.

If you are undergoing a joint replacement, there are two issues to consider:

1. Should the procedure be done as an outpatient?
2. Should it be done at a free-standing surgi-center?

These are complex issues that are controversial and go beyond the scope of this book. But in a nutshell, the biggest factor being debated is safety: what are the odds of a given patient having this or that complication (cardiac/respiratory issues, infections, etc.)? Where are the risks of sustaining these complications lowest (hospital or surgi-center)—or are they the same? Where is it best for a patient to be if a complication does develop—or does it not matter?

A major issue in my opinion is the choice the surgeon has to make between performing the procedure in a hospital or in his/her surgi-center. That involves a judgment call, and that judgment can be clouded by financial gain.

And the final point I wish to bring up takes us back to Chapter 1: the orthopedist has to decide whether you need a procedure in the first place. Can the facility fee be an even more powerful inducement for unnecessary surgery than the surgical fee? Let's see what the future brings.

Index

A

Abductors, 180
Adductors, 180
ACI, 121
ACL, 53
AMZ, 119
Anesthesia, 30
Anterior Knee Pain, 105
Anterior cruciate ligament (ACL), 53
Apley grind, 27
Arthritis, 8, 13, 20, 22, 24, 42, 54, 55, 65, 75–103, 120
Arthroscopy, 30
Aspiration, 174
Autologous Chondrocyte Implantation, 121
Avascular necrosis, 142

B

Baker's cyst, 11, 124
Balance, 181
Bone bruise, 57
Bone on bone, 102
Bone-patella-bone ACL graft, 59, 71
Bucket handle tear, 23–26
Bursitis, 140

C

Cartilage (articular), 8
Cartilage (torn), 4, 10–13, 21–42
Chondromalacia, 105–132
Chondrocalcinosis, 10, 148
Cleavage tear, 24
Cold (treatment), 35
Consequential injury, 201
Core insufficiency/control, 115, 137
CRPS, 138

D

Denervation, 120
Discoid meniscus, 35
Distal re-alignment, 116

E

Effusion, 123,124
Elmslie-Trillat, 118
Exercise, 33, 62, 80, 87–89, 99, 114, 165–194
Extensor mechanism, 109

F

Fat pad, 136
Fibular collateral ligament, 44, 63
Flap tear, 40, 42
Fraud, 195–198
Fulkerson, 119–120

G

Growth plate, 58, 119
Geniculate vessels, 117
Gout, 141

H

Hamstrings, 52, 61, 177, 180–194
Hamstring (ACL) graft, 61
Hauser operation, 116
Heat (treatment), 35

I

Iliotibial band, ITB, 133–135, 144, 166, 173, 190
Informed consent, 77, 140

J

Jumper's knee, 171

K

Kissing lesion, 102

L

Lateral retinaculum, 109,112, 114, 116–117, 120
Laser, 29
Lateral collateral ligament, 44, 63
Lateral release, 116–118
Locking, 26, 28
Lupus, 141
Lyme, 141

M

Maquet, 123
McMurray, 26
Medial collateral ligament, 44–52, 170–174
Meniscal tears (types), 21–42
Microfracture, 121
MRI (torn cartilage), 21–42
MRI misleading, 7–20, 123, 145, 147–148
Malalignment (kneecap), 8, 9, 109, 110
McMurray, 26
Merchant (x-ray view), 77, 112, 116, 147, 149, 153
Merchant, Alan, 77

N

Neuroma, 136–137, 196
Neuritis, 117

O
OATS, 121
Osgood-Schlatter, 140
OCD (osteochondritis dissecans), 142
Osteochondromatosis, 142

P
Parrot-beak tear, 24
Partial knee replacement, 93, 121
Patella alta, 118–120, 140
Patella baja, 118
Patellofemoral syndrome, 105
Patellar tendon, 59–61, 108–109, 117, 119, 127
Patellectomy, 121
Patellofemoral replacement, 94, 121
PCL, 44, 63
Physical therapy, 87, 95, 99, 105–106, 110, 113–114
Pigmented villonodular synovitis (PVNS), 142
Placebo, 13, 155
Placebo reverse/ MRI, 141
Pool, 34, 89, 183–184
Posterior cruciate ligament, 44, 63
Proximal re-alignment, 116
Psoriatic arthritis, 141

Q
Q angle, 109, 118–119, 127
Quadriceps, 59–61, 108–109
Quadriceps tendon, 59–60

R
Racquetball, 169
Radial tear, 40
Referred pain, 139
Reflex Sympathetic Dystrophy, 138
Reiter's syndrome, 141
Rheumatism, 141
Rheumatoid arthritis, 141
Rosenberg x-ray view, 78, 146
RSD, 138
Runner's knee, 134, 144
Running, 62, 89, 135, 166

S
Sciatica, 189
Shoes, 89, 96, 98, 135
Signal change (on an MRI), 10
Standing flexion x-ray view, 146
Stem cells, 97, 121
Stretching, 99, 114, 134, 167, 169, 171, 175–177
Strengthening, 34–35, 87, 179
Synovitis, 36, 38, 142
Synovium, 38, 143

T

Tendinitis, 23, 88, 97, 134, 166, 173
Tendinitis (patellar), 97, 135
Tendinosis, 136
Tennis, 169–170
Terrible triad, 170
Tibial tuberosity, 60, 116, 118–120, 140
Torn Cartilage , 4, 8, 10–13, 21
Trick knee, 53, 56
Trochlea, 108–128, 147, 152
Tumors, 122, 143
Tunnel x-ray view, 146

V

VMO, 95, 180, 126

W

Wall slides, 34, 180
Water exercises, 89, 96, 183
Women, 55, 142, 171

About the Author

Ronald Grelsamer, MD is an orthopedic surgeon in New York City affiliated with the Icahn School of Medicine at the Mount Sinai Medical Center. He has over ninety publications to his name and consults on knee and hip issues out of his private office in Manhattan.

See his website, www.rpgOrtho.com, for further details.